**Questions and Answers in
Oral Health Education**

Questions and Answers in Oral Health Education

Chloe Foxhall
RDN cert OHE cert RAD cert IQA PTLLS
Registered Dental Nurse working for a mixed NHS and Private practice
Dental Tutor for Smiles Dental Training LTD
Internal Quality Assurance

Anna Lown
RDN LCGI cert OHE cert IQA PTLLS
Registered Dental Nurse
Founder and Director of Smiles Dental Training LTD
Dental Tutor and Assessor
Internal Quality Assurance
Level 3 Certificate in Assessing Vocational Achievement

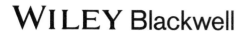

WILEY Blackwell

This edition first published 2021
© 2021 John Wiley & Sons Ltd

The right of Chloe Foxhall and Anna Lown to be identified as the authors of this work has been asserted in accordance with law.

Registered Offices
John Wiley & Sons, Inc., 111 River Street, Hoboken, NJ 07030, USA
John Wiley & Sons Ltd, The Atrium, Southern Gate, Chichester, West Sussex, PO19 8SQ, UK

Editorial Office
9600 Garsington Road, Oxford, OX4 2DQ, UK

For details of our global editorial offices, customer services, and more information about Wiley products visit us at www.wiley.com.

Wiley also publishes its books in a variety of electronic formats and by print-on-demand. Some content that appears in standard print versions of this book may not be available in other formats.

Library of Congress Cataloging-in-Publication Data

Names: Foxhall, Chloe, author. | Lown, Anna, author.
Title: Questions and answers in oral health education / Chloe Foxhall, Anna
    Lown.
Description: Hoboken, NJ : Wiley-Blackwell, 2021. | Includes
    bibliographical references.
Identifiers: LCCN 2020030616 (print) | LCCN 2020030617 (ebook) |
    ISBN 9781119647270 (paperback) | ISBN 9781119647256 (adobe pdf) |
    ISBN 9781119647300 (epub)
Subjects: MESH: Oral Health | Mouth Diseases | Health Education, Dental |
    Examination Questions
Classification: LCC RK307 (print) | LCC RK307 (ebook) | NLM WU 18.2 |
    DDC 616.3/1–dc23
LC record available at https://lccn.loc.gov/2020030616
LC ebook record available at https://lccn.loc.gov/2020030617

Cover Design: Wiley
Cover Image: Courtesy of Chloe Foxhall

Set in 9.5/12.5pt STIXTwoText by SPi Global, Pondicherry, India
Printed and bound by CPI Group (UK) Ltd, Croydon, CR0 4YY

10 9 8 7 6 5 4 3 2 1

To Pieter Roos and Niel Pienaar for allowing us the opportunity to begin our careers in dentistry. For their love, support, and encouragement, we will be forever thankful.

Contents

Acknowledgements

Chloe Foxhall

To my partner, Chas Stephenson, who continues to love and support me throughout all of my personal and professional challenges.

To my parents, family, and friends, for always being there for me with reassurance and continuous support with everything I do, especially my mother who has given her time to read and correct my grammar while writing this book.

A heartfelt thank you to my colleague and friend Anna Lown who has supported me as a tutor and dental nurse and has taken her time to work alongside me on this book. I am truly grateful for the opportunity.

Anna Lown

To my husband Bobie and son Chester, for the love and support which they have given me to be able to help write this book. To my parents and family, for their encouragement throughout my career as a dental nurse and dental tutor, and for always being there for me.

I would also like to thank colleagues and work friends who make dentistry and teaching so enjoyable and gratifying.

Without a doubt, I would like to thank all of the dental practices and students who have used, and continue to use, us at Smiles Dental Training Ltd as their chosen course provider. For putting their trust in us to help them achieve their goals and start or progress in their career in dentistry.

Lastly, thank you to my colleague and friend Chloe, who had a dream about collaborating and writing a book together, and who helped turn that dream into a reality. Whoever would have thought that we would be where we are now! I thank you for everything.

From us both:

Finally, a special thank you to Wiley Blackwell for publishing this book. A dream has been made into a reality to support other dental professionals in oral health education.

About the Authors

Chloe Foxhall

Chloe is a qualified dental nurse and holds postgraduate certificates in Oral Health Education and Radiography as well as a L3 in Education and Training and L4 Internal Quality Assurance. She works as a dental nurse in a general dental practice and as a dental tutor for Smiles Dental Training Ltd. Chloe has written various continuing professional development courses for a range of topics, including safeguarding and mental capacity.

She enjoys shopping, travel, and reading. Chloe likes to take on new challenges by learning about different subjects based around dentistry.

Anna Lown

Anna is a director of her own Company, Smiles Dental Training Ltd, a training company specialising in dental nurse training and education. She holds postgraduate certificates in Oral Health Education and Topical Fluoride Application as well as PTLLS, Certificate in Assessing Vocational Achievement, and L4 IQA certificates in Education. Anna is a registered dental nurse and holds a City and Guilds Licentiateship in Dental Nursing. She works as the director of Smiles Dental Training Ltd and as a dental tutor/assessor.

Anna has written NEBDN training courses as well as CPD courses for other companies. She has also been involved with course development and oral health education for other healthcare sectors.

She enjoys family holidays in the Lake District, hiking, and reading.

Anna welcomes any comments or interest from readers. Please contact her via her website: www.smilesdentaltraining.co.uk

Introduction

This book is designed to be an invaluable revision tool to assist students who are undertaking their Certificate in Oral Health Education and help to prepare them for their upcoming exam.

It provides an outline of the core topics that an oral health educator would be expected to have knowledge and understanding of and should be used as a revision tool alongside lecture notes and textbooks relating to oral health education. This book is intended as a resource to test the level of knowledge and understanding, while giving in-depth descriptions of the correct answers for each question. It also demonstrates multiple choice questions and extended matching question formats to help preparation for the final exam.

The book contains chapters on areas such as Oral Health Messages, Anatomy and the Oral Mucosa, Sugars, Lesson Preparation, and Communication. The wide range of topics covered will help underpin the knowledge required to be able to successfully pass the oral health education exam. It has been carefully designed to be easy to use through separating each topic into revision sections, which are then divided into question and answer format.

We hope that this book provides guidance and support to you during your studies and we thank you as our readers and students. We wish you all the best in your dental career.

How to use Question and Answers in Oral Health Education

This book has been written based on two styles of questions: multiple choice questions and extended matching questions that are used in the National Examination Board for Dental Nurses (NEBDN) Post Registration Qualification in Oral Health Education exam. Students should read through this section of the book before using it as a revision guide in order to gain the best possible understanding of how the questions are prepared.

This book is designed to aid revision for students wanting to progress their knowledge in oral health education.

Multiple Choice Questions (MCQ)

Multiple choice questions are usually a one- or two-line question that has several possible answers. They usually will provide some subject matter in the first line and the second line will ask the question; sometimes these will be combined. The answers will be written in alphabetical or numerical order and only one answer will be correct. Each question is worth one mark.

All of the questions are written in the same format; therefore, the student will need to have the relevant knowledge to apply to the scenario of the question in order to answer it correctly and score one mark.

During the exam, the student will have a marking sheet on which their answers should be marked in pencil with a single horizontal line through the appropriate square. Only one box should be marked for each question otherwise the computer marking system will reject the student's answer for that question and will leave the student without a mark. The marking system will also reject any question that is marked with a cross (x), a tick (✓), or a circle (O).

Extended Matching Questions (EMQ)

Extended matching questions are in the same format as the multiple choice questions; however, the student is often given a scenario to provide background information, and then follows the question. There are a minimum of six answers to choose from, usually at least 8, and the same option list is used for at least two questions. Each of the lists of answers are based around one topic.

The student will mark the answers on a marking sheet in pencil with a single horizontal line through the appropriate square. Only one box should be marked for each question otherwise the computer marking system will reject the student's answer for that question and leave the student without a mark. The marking system will also reject any question that is marked with a cross (x), a tick (✓), or a circle (O).

All of the questions are written in the same format; therefore, the student will need to have the relevant knowledge to apply to the scenario of the question in order to answer it correctly and score one mark.

About the Companion Website

This book also has a companion website:

www.wiley.com/go/foxhall/oral-health-education

This website includes:

- Multiple choice questions
- Extended matching questions
- Sample questions and keywords
- Videos

Roles and Responsibilities

In a dental practice there are many people that make up a team in order to have a well functioning unit. This includes dentists, hygienists, therapists, and dental nurses. Clinicians are able to take on further studies and become specialists in various other fields, such as oral surgery or endodontics. Dental Care Professionals (DCPs) are now able to study to hold extended duties. Some examples of these are oral health education, radiography, sedation nursing, impression taking, or implant nursing.

Dentist

A student spends five years completing undergraduate training at a university dental school. When the final examinations are completed, the students are awarded a Bachelor of Dental Surgery (BDS) which then allows them to enrol onto the dentist register with the General Dental Council (GDC). The register is held by the GDC and contains the dentist's full name, GDC number, and qualifications; the register is made public so patients can access these details.

Dentists that are registered have many opportunities to progress in the profession depending on their interests. Some of the options they have depending on location are:

- general practice, either NHS or private
- community dental services
- educational services
- armed forces
- hospital services.

Dental Nurse

A dental nurse is trained to work alongside the dentist and support them while servicing patients in whichever area they decide to work; this could be in a general practice, NHS, or private, community dental services, armed forces, or hospital services. Before 2008, dental nurses were not classed as a registered profession. A dental nurse at that time could be recruited and work without any education or professional qualification. Now, a dental nurse – on completing their qualification with an accredited course provider – must register with the GDC in order to continue working. This registration is then renewed every year in order to continue working in the profession.

A dental nurse role should include, but is not limited to, the following:

- Performing chairside assistance to a dentist, hygienist, or therapist throughout all procedures safely and effectively and in accordance to the GDCS scope of practice and your level of training.
- Following practice policies and procedures.
- Maintaining indemnity and registration with the GDC.
- Undertaking CPD in line with the GDC guidelines for E-CPD.
- Maintaining and promoting productive working relationships with colleagues.
- Assisting any trainee dental nurses within the practice.
- Assisting with any reception or other clerical duties as required.
- Following health and safety guidelines to ensure safety for all members of the dental team.
- Complying with all guidelines, such as: PPE, COSHH, mercury handling, infection control, and waste disposal.
- Acting in accordance to all practice rules and codes of conduct.

Key tasks for a dental nurse could be, but are not limited to:

- Following the practice procedures for infection prevention and control.
- Setting up and preparing treatment rooms for each patient's appointment.
- Preparing necessary materials and instruments, making sure that equipment and instruments are in safe working order.
- Disposing of waste in the correct bins, such as clinical waste, special waste, and normal waste.
- Assisting during taking and development of radiographs to your level of training.
- Having relevant paperwork ready on reception, in surgery, or for a patient if requested.
- Preparing and sending referrals to your level of training.
- Maintaining and decontaminating equipment as per manufacturer's instructions.
- Providing chairside support to the dentist, hygienist, or therapist during treatments.
- Preparing materials and equipment.
- Assisting in keeping full, accurate, and contemporaneous clinical notes for each patient.
- Monitoring, supporting, and reassuring patients.
- Supporting colleagues if there is a medical emergency.
- Following all compliance rules set out by your practice.

Oral Health Educator

An oral health educator has an important role within the dental setting to help prevent oral disease and promote good oral healthcare. Working as an educator means you have to hold a session, seeing patients on a one-to-one basis and promoting good oral health. These sessions could be held with a range of patients from children right the way through to senior patients. You may even be required to work within the community, meeting at schools and providing group sessions offering advice to children and their parents. As an oral health educator, you may want to expand your knowledge onto further areas such as:

- diet and nutrition
- impression taking
- fluoride application
- smoking cessation.

Working as an oral health educator, you are aiming to:

- Reduce the patient's risk of dental caries, periodontal disease, and oral cancer.
- Improve the patient's quality of life, including social and mental wellbeing.
- Improve the patient's education on how to care for their oral health.

To complete the aims outlined above, you may be asked to:

- Give advice to patients within a dental practice setting on referral from a dentist or orthodontist.
- Travel out into the community to visit schools, care homes, foster homes, etc.
- Provide group educational sessions to a certain target group.
- Provide oral health instructions while working under supervision of a dentist.
- Support clinical public health programmes/projects.
- Participate in the design, development, and maintenance of oral health education materials, equipment, and visual aids.
- Deliver in-service training for healthcare/multiagency staff and to the staff in educational establishments.

Standards for the Dental Team – GDC

The GDC created the Standards for the Dental Team in 2013. They were put in place so dental care professionals have a strong understanding of what is expected of them within their role. The document contains nine principles; each principle outlines the patient's expectation, and the standards and the guidance on how this should be achieved and maintained day to day. The document clearly states that the nine principles are not placed in order of importance or priority. The standards that fall under each principle are what **must** be followed. The guidance is given to help meet the standards. All dental care professionals are expected to follow the guidance to provide professional judgements where necessary; if judgement is made, it should be easily justifiable if it is not in line with the guidance given. Within the document, anything that **should** be applied, may not apply to every situation through exceptional circumstances – which is when your judgement on how to handle the situation would be taken into account.

Principle 1 – Put Patients' Interests First

Patient expectation:

- To be able to explain preferences or concerns to a professional who will listen and take all information into consideration.
- To be able to express their cultures and values within the practice and be respected as an individual.
- That all professionals will work honestly and with integrity.
- To receive treatment from a plan that has been created for the individual in accordance with the patient's health and wellbeing.
- That the environment is clean and safe.
- To be able to access the practice by reasonable adjustment if the patient has a disability.
- That financial gain will not be the top priority and the patient's needs will always be put first.
- If any harm is suffered during dental treatment, then the staff will redress this.
- That any pain or anxiety that could be experienced will be managed as required.

The following information has been extracted from the GDC Standards for the Dental Team document.

Standard 1.1 Listen to your patients
1.1.1 You must provide the patient with a full discussion on the treatment options and listen carefully to anything the patient may disclose. Welcome questions from the patient.

Standard 1.2 Treat every patient with dignity and respect at all times
1.2.1 Your body language and tone of voice should be considered on how it may be perceived.
1.2.2 You should take patients' preferences into account and be sensitive to their individual needs and values.
1.2.3 You must treat patients with kindness and compassion.
1.2.4 You should manage patients' dental pain and anxiety appropriately, to ensure the comfort of the patient being treated.

Standard 1.3 Be honest and act with integrity
1.3.1 You must justify the trust that patients, the public, and your colleagues place in you by always acting honestly and fairly in your dealings with them. This applies to any business or education activities in which you are involved as well as to your professional dealings.
1.3.2 You must make sure you do not bring the profession to disrepute.
1.3.3 You must make sure that any advertising, promotional material, or other information that you produce is accurate and not misleading and complies with the GDC's guidance on ethical advertising.

Standard 1.4 Take a holistic and preventative approach to patient care which is appropriate to the individual patient

1.4.1 A holistic approach means you must take account of patients' overall health, their psychological, and social needs, their long term oral health needs, and their desired outcomes.

1.4.2 You must provide patients with treatment that is in their best interests, providing appropriate oral health advice and following clinical guidelines relevant to their situation. You may need to balance their oral health needs with their desired outcomes. If their desired outcome is not achievable or is not in the best interests of their oral health, you must explain the risks, benefits, and likely outcomes to help them to make a decision.

Standard 1.5 Treat patients in a hygienic and safe environment

1.5.1 You must find out about the laws and regulations which apply to your clinical practice, your premises, and your obligations as an employer and you must follow them at all times. This will include (but is not limited to) legislation relating to:

- the disposal of clinical and other hazardous waste
- radiography
- health and safety
- decontamination
- medical devices.

1.5.2 You must make sure that you have all necessary vaccinations and follow guidance relating to blood-borne viruses.

1.5.3 You must follow the guidance on medical emergencies and training updates issued by the Resuscitation Council (UK).

1.5.4 You must record all patient safety incidents and report them promptly to the appropriate national body.

Standard 1.6 Treat patients fairly, as individuals, and without discrimination

1.6.1 You must not discriminate against patients on the grounds of:

- age
- disability
- gender reassignment
- marriage and civil partnership
- pregnancy and maternity
- race
- religion or belief
- sex
- sexual orientation.

You must also ensure that you do not discriminate against patients or groups of patients for any other reasons such as nationality, special needs, health, lifestyle, or any other consideration.

1.6.2 You must be aware of and adhere to all your responsibilities as set out in relevant equalities legislation.

1.6.3 You must consider patients' disabilities and make reasonable adjustments to allow them to receive care which meets their needs. If you cannot make reasonable adjustments to treat a patient safely, you should consider referring them to a colleague.

1.6.4 You must not express your personal beliefs (including political, religious, or moral beliefs) to patients in any way that exploits their vulnerability or could cause them distress.

Standard 1.7 Put patients' interest before your own boss or those of any colleague, business, or organisation.

1.7.1 You must always put your patients' interests before any financial, personal, or other gain.

1.7.2 If you work in a practice that provides both NHS (or equivalent health service) and private treatment (a mixed practice), you must make clear to your patients which treatments can be provided under the NHS (or equivalent health service) and which can only be provided on a private basis.

1.7.3 You must not mislead patients into believing that treatments which are available on the NHS (or equivalent health service) can only be provided privately. If you work in a purely private practice, you should make sure that patients know this before they attend for treatment.

1.7.4 If you work in a mixed practice, you must not pressurise patients into having private treatment if it is available to them under the NHS (or equivalent health service) and they would prefer to have it under the NHS (or equivalent health service).

1.7.5 You must refuse any gifts, payment, or hospitality if accepting them could affect, or could appear to affect, your professional judgement.

1.7.6 When you are referring patients to another member of the dental team, you must make sure that the referral is made in the patients' best interests rather than for your own, or another team member's, financial gain or benefit.

1.7.7 If you believe that patients might be at risk because of your health, behaviour, or professional performance or that of a colleague, or because of any aspect of the clinical environment, you must take prompt and appropriate action.

1.7.8 In rare circumstances, the trust between you and a patient may break down, and you may find it necessary to end the professional relationship. You should not stop providing a service to a patient solely because of a complaint the patient has made about you or your team. Before you end a professional relationship with a patient, you must be satisfied that your decision is fair and you must be able to justify your decision. You should write to the patient to tell them your decision and your reasons for it. You should take steps to ensure that arrangements are made promptly for the continuing care of the patient.

Standard 1.8 Have appropriate arrangement in place for patients to seek compensation if they suffer harm

1.8.1 You must have appropriate insurance or indemnity in place to make sure your patients can claim any compensation to which they may be entitled.

1.8.2 You should ensure that you keep to the terms and conditions of your insurance or indemnity and contact the provider as soon as possible when a claim is made. A delay in contacting the provider could disadvantage patients and may affect the level of help you receive from the provider.

Standard 1.9 Find out about laws and regulations that affect your work and follow them.

1.9.1 You must find out about, and follow, laws and regulations affecting your work. This includes, but is not limited to, those relating to:

- data protection
- employment
- human rights and equality
- registration with other regulatory bodies.

Principle 2 – Communicate Effectively with Patients

Patient expectation:

- To receive full, clear, and accurate information that they can understand, before, during, and after treatment, so that they can make informed decisions in partnership with the people providing their care.
- A clear explanation of the treatment, possible outcomes and what they can expect.
- To know how much their treatment will cost before it starts, and to be told about any changes.
- Communication that they can understand.
- To know the names of those providing their care.

Standard 2.1 Communicate effectively with patients – listen to them, give them time to consider information, and take their individual views and communication needs into account.

2.1.1 You must treat patients as individuals. You should take their specific communication needs and preferences into account where possible and respect any cultural values and differences.

2.1.2 You must be sufficiently fluent in written and spoken English to communicate effectively with patients, their relatives, the dental team, and other healthcare professionals in the United Kingdom.

Standard 2.2 Recognise and promote patients' rights to and responsibilities for making decisions about their health priorities and care.

2.2.1 You must listen to patients and communicate effectively with them at a level they can understand. Before treatment starts you must:
- explain the options (including those of delaying treatment or doing nothing) with the risks and benefits of each; and
- give full information on the treatment you propose and the possible costs.

2.2.2 You should encourage patients to ask questions about their options or any aspect of their treatment.

2.2.3 You must give full and honest answers to any questions patients have about their options or treatment.

Standard 2.3 Give patients the information they need, in a way they can understand, so that they can make informed decisions.

2.3.1 You should introduce yourself to patients and explain your role so that they know how you will be involved in their care.

2.3.2 Other members of your team may have valuable knowledge about the patients' backgrounds or concerns so you should involve them (and the patients' carers if relevant) in discussion with patients where appropriate.

2.3.3 You should recognise patients' communication difficulties and try to meet the patients' particular communication needs by, for example:

- not using professional jargon and acronyms;
- using an interpreter for patients whose first language is not English;
- suggesting that patients bring someone with them who can use sign language; and
- providing an induction loop to help patients who wear hearing aids.

2.3.4 You should satisfy yourself that patients have understood the information you have given them, for example by asking questions and summarising the main points of your discussion.

2.3.5 You should make sure that patients have enough information and enough time to ask questions and make a decision.

2.3.6 You must give patients a written treatment plan, or plans, before their treatment starts and you should retain a copy in their notes. You should also ask patients to sign the treatment plan.

2.3.7 Whenever you provide a treatment plan you must include:

- the proposed treatment;
- a realistic indication of the cost;
- whether the treatment is being provided under the NHS (or equivalent health service) or privately (if mixed, the treatment plan should clearly indicate which elements are being provided under which arrangement).

2.3.8 You should keep the treatment plan and estimated costs under review during treatment. You must inform your patients immediately if the treatment plan changes and provide them with an updated version in writing.

2.3.9 You must provide patients with clear information about your arrangements for emergency care including the out of hours arrangements.

2.3.10 You should make sure patients have the details they need to allow them to contact you by their preferred method.

2.3.11 You should provide patients with clear information about any referral arrangements related to their treatment.

Standard 2.4 Give patients clear information about costs.

2.4.1 You must make sure that a simple price list is clearly displayed in your reception or waiting area. This should include a list of basic items including a consultation, a single-surface filling, an extraction, radiographs (bitewing or pan-oral) and treatment provided by the hygienist. For items which may vary in cost, a 'from–to' price range can be shown.

2.4.2 You must give clear information on prices in your practice literature and on your websites – patients should not have to ask for this information.

2.4.3 You should tell your patients whether treatment is guaranteed, under what circumstances and for how long. You should make clear any circumstances under which treatment is not guaranteed (for example, a lack of care on their part which leads to recurring problems).

Principle 3 – Obtain Valid Consent

Patient expectation:

- To be asked for their consent to treatment before it starts.

Standard 3.1 Obtain valid consent before starting treatment, explaining all the relevant options and the possible costs.

3.1.1 You must make sure you have valid consent before starting any treatment or investigation. This applies whether you are the first member of your team to see the patient or whether you are involved after other team members have already seen them. Do not assume that someone else has obtained the patient's consent.

3.1.2 You should document the discussions you have with patients in the process of gaining consent. Although a signature on a form is important in verifying that a patient has given consent, it is the discussions that take place with the patient that determine whether the consent is valid.

3.1.3 You should find out what your patients want to know as well as what you think they need to know. Things that patients might want to know include:

- options for treatment, the risks, and the potential benefits;
- why you think a particular treatment is necessary and appropriate for them;
- the consequences, risks, and benefits of the treatment you propose;
- the likely prognosis;
- your recommended option;
- the cost of the proposed treatment;
- what might happen if the proposed treatment is not carried out; and
- whether the treatment is guaranteed, how long it is guaranteed for and any exclusions that apply.

3.1.4 You must check and document that patients have understood the information you have given.

3.1.5 Patients can withdraw their consent at any time, refuse treatment, or ask for it to be stopped after it has started. You must acknowledge their right to do this and follow their wishes. You should explain the consequences or risks of not continuing the treatment and ensure that the patient knows that they are responsible for any future problems which arise as a result of not completing the treatment. You must record all this in the patient's notes.

3.1.6 You must obtain written consent where treatment involves conscious sedation or general anaesthetic.

Standard 3.2 Make sure that patients (or their representatives) understand the decisions they are being asked to make.

3.2.1 You must provide patients with sufficient information and give them a reasonable amount of time to consider that information in order to make a decision.

3.2.2 You must tailor the way you obtain consent to each patient's needs. You should help them to make informed decisions about their care by giving them information in a format they can easily understand.

3.2.3 When obtaining consent, you should encourage patients who have communication difficulties to have a friend, relative, or carer with them to help them ask questions or understand your answers.

3.2.4 You must always consider whether patients are able to make decisions about their care themselves, and avoid making assumptions about a patient's ability to give consent.

3.2.5 You must check and document that patients have understood the information you have given them.

Standard 3.3 Make sure that the patient's consent remains valid at each stage of investigation or treatment.

3.3.1 Giving and obtaining consent is a process, not a one-off event. It should be part of ongoing communication between patients and all members of the dental team involved in their care. You should keep patients informed about the progress of their care.

3.3.2 When carrying out an ongoing course of treatment, you must make sure you have specific consent for what you are going to do during that appointment.

3.3.3 You must tailor the way you confirm ongoing consent to each patient's needs and check that patients have understood the information you have given them.

3.3.4 You must document the discussions you have with patients in the process of confirming their ongoing consent.

3.3.5 If you think that you need to change a patient's agreed treatment or the estimated cost, you must obtain your patient's consent to the changes and document that you have done so.

Principle 4 – Maintain and Protect Patients' Information

Patient expectation:

- Their records to be up to date, complete, clear, accurate, and legible.
- Their personal details to be kept confidential.
- To be able to access their dental records.
- Their records to be stored securely.

Standard 4.1 Make and keep contemporaneous, complete and accurate patient records.

4.1.1 You must make and keep complete and accurate patient records, including an up-to-date medical history, each time that you treat patients. Radiographs, consent forms, photographs, models, audio or visual recordings of consultations, laboratory prescriptions, statements of conformity, and referral letters all form part of patients' records where they are available.

4.1.2 You should record as much detail as possible about the discussions you have with your patients, including evidence that valid consent has been obtained. You should also include details of any particular patient's treatment needs where appropriate.

4.1.3 You must understand and meet your responsibilities in relation to patient information in line with current legislation. You must follow appropriate national advice on retaining, storing, and disposing of patient records.

4.1.4 You must ensure that all documentation that records your work, including patient records, is clear, legible, accurate, and can be readily understood by others. You must also record the name or initials of the treating clinician.

4.1.5 If you need to make any amendments to a patient's records, you must make sure that the changes are clearly marked up and dated.

4.1.6 If you refer a patient to another dental professional or other health professional, you must make an accurate record of this referral in the patient's notes and include a written prescription when necessary.

Standard 4.2 Protect the confidentiality of patients' information and only use it for the purpose for which it was given.

4.2.1 Confidentiality is central to the relationship and trust between you and your patients. You must keep patient information confidential. This applies to all the information about patients that you have learnt in your professional role including personal details, medical history, what treatment they are having, and how much it costs.

4.2.2 You must ensure that non-registered members of the dental team are aware of the importance of confidentiality and that they keep patient information confidential at all times.

4.2.3 You must not post any information or comments about patients on social networking or blogging sites. If you use professional social media to discuss anonymised cases for the purpose of discussing best practice, you must be careful that the patient or patients cannot be identified.

4.2.4 You must not talk about patients or their treatment in places where you can be overheard by people who should not have access to the information you are discussing.

4.2.5 You must explain to patients the circumstances in which you may need to share information with others involved in their healthcare. This includes making sure that they understand:

- what information you will be releasing;
- why you will be releasing it; and
- the likely consequences of you releasing the information. You must give your patients the opportunity to withhold their permission to share information in this way unless exceptional circumstances apply. You must record in your patient's notes whether or not they gave their permission.

4.2.6 If a patient allows you to share information about them, you should ensure that anyone you share it with understands that it is confidential.

4.2.7 If other people ask you to provide information about patients (for example, for teaching or research), or if you want to use patient information such as photographs for any reason, you must:

- explain to patients how the information or images will be used;
- check that patients understand what they are agreeing to;
- obtain and record the patients' consent to their use;
- only release or use the minimum information necessary for the purpose; and
- explain to the patients that they can withdraw their permission at any time. If it is not necessary for patients to be identified, you must make sure they remain anonymous in any information you release.

4.2.8 You must keep patient information confidential even after patients die.

4.2.9 The duty to keep information confidential also covers recordings or images of patients such as photographs, videos, or audio recordings, both originals and copies, including those made on a mobile phone. You must not make any recordings or images without the patient's permission.

Standard 4.3 Only release a patient's information without their permission in exceptional circumstances.

4.3.1 In exceptional circumstances, you may be justified in releasing confidential patient information without their consent if doing so is in the best interests of the public or the patient. This could happen if a patient puts their own safety or that of others at serious risk, or if information about a patient could be important in preventing or detecting a serious crime.

If you believe that revealing information about a patient is in the best interests of the public or the patient, you should first try to get the patient's permission to release the information.

You should do everything you can to encourage the patient to either release the information themselves or to give you permission to do so. You must document the efforts you have made to obtain consent in the patient's notes.

4.3.2 If obtaining consent from a patient to the release of their information in the public interest is not practical or appropriate, or if the patient will not give their permission, you should get advice from your defence organisation or professional association before you release the information.

4.3.3 If you have information that a patient is or could be at risk of significant harm, or you suspect that a patient is a victim of abuse, you must inform the appropriate social care agencies or the police.

4.3.4 You can be ordered by a court, or you can be under a statutory duty, to release information about a patient without their permission. If this happens, you should only release the minimum amount of information necessary to comply with the court order or statutory duty.

4.3.5 In any circumstance where you decide to release confidential information, you must document your reasons and be prepared to explain and justify your decision and actions.

Standard 4.4 Ensure that patients can have access to their records.

4.4.1 Although patients do not own their dental records, they have the right to access them under Data Protection legislation. If patients ask for access to their records, you must arrange for this promptly, in accordance with the law.

4.4.2 In some circumstances you can charge patients a fee for accessing their records. The maximum you can charge depends on whether the records are paper copies or held electronically. You should check the latest guidance issued by your national Information Commissioner's Office.

Standard 4.5 Keep patients' information secure at all times, whether your records are held on paper or electronically.

4.5.1 You must make sure that patients' information is not revealed accidentally and that no one has unauthorised access to it by storing it securely at all times. You must not leave records where they can be seen by other patients, unauthorised staff or members, or the public.

4.5.2 If you are sending confidential information, you should use a secure method. If you are sending or storing confidential information electronically, you should ensure that it is encrypted.

4.5.3 If clinical records are computerised, you should make back-up copies of clinical records, radiographs, and other images.

Principle 5 – Have a Clear and Effective Complaints Procedure

Patient expectations:

• Their concerns or complaints to be acknowledged, listened to, and dealt with promptly.

Standard 5.1 Make sure that there is an effective complaints procedure readily available for patients to use and follow that procedure at all times.

5.1.1 It is part of your responsibility as a dental professional to deal with complaints properly and professionally. You must:

• ensure that there is an effective written complaints procedure where you work;
• follow the complaints procedure at all times;
• respond to complaints within the time limits set out in the procedure; and
• provide a constructive response to the complaint.

5.1.2 You should make sure that everyone (dental professionals, other staff, and patients) knows about the complaints procedure and understands how it works. If you are an employer, or you manage a team, you must ensure that all staff are trained in handling complaints.

5.1.3 If you work for a practice that provides NHS (or equivalent health service) treatment, or if you work in a hospital, you should follow the procedure set down by that organisation.

5.1.4 If you work in private practice, including private practice owned by a dental body corporate, you should make sure that it has a procedure which sets similar standards and time limits to the NHS (or equivalent health service) procedure.

5.1.5 You should make sure that your complaints procedure:

- is displayed where patients can see it – patients should not have to ask for a copy;
- is clearly written in plain language and is available in other formats if needed;
- is easy for patients to understand and follow;
- provides information on other independent organisations that patients can contact to raise concerns;
- allows you to deal with complaints promptly and efficiently;
- allows you to investigate complaints in a full and fair way;
- explains the possible outcomes;
- allows information that can be used to improve services to pass back to your practice management or equivalent; and
- respects patients' confidentiality.

5.1.6 Complaints can be an opportunity to improve your service. You should analyse any complaints that you receive to help you improve the service you offer, and share lessons learnt from complaints with all team members.

5.1.7 You should keep a written record of all complaints together with your responses. This record should be separate from your patient records so that patients are not discouraged from making a complaint.

You should use your record of complaints to monitor your performance in handling complaints and identify any areas that need to be improved.

Standard 5.2 Respect a patient's right to complain.

5.2.1 You should not react defensively to complaints. You should listen carefully to patients who complain and involve them fully in the complaints process. You should find out what outcome patients want from their complaint.

Standard 5.3 Give patients who complain a prompt and constructive response.

5.3.1 You should give the patient a copy of the complaints procedure when you acknowledge their complaint so that they understand the stages involved and the timescales.

5.3.2 You should deal with complaints in a calm and constructive way and in line with the complaints procedure.

5.3.3 You should aim to resolve complaints as efficiently, effectively, and politely as possible.

5.3.4 You must respond to complaints within the time limits set out in your complaints procedure.

5.3.5 If you need more time to investigate a complaint, you should tell the patient when you will respond.

5.3.6 If there are exceptional circumstances which mean that the complaint cannot be resolved within the usual timescale, you should give the patient regular updates (at least every 10 days) on progress.

5.3.7 You should try to deal with all the points raised in the complaint and, where possible, offer a solution for each one.

5.3.8 You should offer an apology and a practical solution where appropriate.

5.3.9 If a complaint is justified, you should offer a fair solution. This may include offering to put things right at your own expense if you have made a mistake.

5.3.10 You should respond to the patient in writing, setting out your findings and any practical solutions you are prepared to offer. Make sure that the letter is clear, deals with the patient's concerns, and is easy for them to understand.

5.3.11 If the patient is not satisfied despite your best efforts to resolve their complaint, you should tell them about other avenues that are open to them, such as the relevant Ombudsman for health service complaints or the Dental Complaints Service for complaints about private dental treatment.

Principle 6 – Work with Colleagues in a Way that Is in the Patient's Best Interest

Patient expectation:

- To be fully informed of the different roles of the dental professionals involved in their care.
- That members of the dental team will work effectively together.

Standard 6.1 Work effectively with your colleagues and contribute to good teamwork.

6.1.1 You should ensure that any team you are involved in works together to provide appropriate dental care for your patients.

6.1.2 You must treat colleagues fairly and with respect, in all situations and all forms of interaction and communication. You must not bully, harass, or unfairly discriminate against them.

6.1.3 You must treat colleagues fairly in all financial transactions.

6.1.4 You must value and respect the contribution of all team members.

6.1.5 You must ensure that patients are fully informed of the names and roles of the dental professionals involved in their care.

6.1.6 As a registered dental professional, you could be held responsible for the actions of any member of your team who does not have to register with the GDC (for example, receptionists, practice managers, or laboratory assistants). You should ensure that they are appropriately trained and competent.

Standard 6.2 Be appropriately supported when treating patients.

6.2.1 You must not provide treatment if you feel that the circumstances make it unsafe for patients.

6.2.2 You should work with another appropriately trained member of the dental team at all times when treating patients in a dental setting. The only circumstances in which this does not apply are when:

- treating patients in an out of hours emergency;
- providing treatment as part of a public health programme; or
- there are exceptional circumstances.

'Exceptional circumstances' are unavoidable circumstances which are not routine and could not have been foreseen. Absences due to leave or training are not exceptional circumstances.

6.2.3 If there are exceptional circumstances which mean you cannot work with an appropriately trained member of the dental team when treating a patient in a dental setting, you must assess the possible risk to the patient of continuing treatment.

6.2.4 If you are providing treatment in a hospital setting, you should be supported by a GDC registrant or a registrant of another healthcare regulator.

6.2.5 If you are providing treatment in a care or domiciliary setting, you should be supported by a GDC registrant or an appropriately trained care professional.

6.2.6 Medical emergencies can happen at any time. You must make sure that there is at least one other person available within the working environment to deal with medical emergencies when you are treating patients. In exceptional circumstances the second person could be a receptionist or a person accompanying the patient.

Standard 6.3 Delegate and refer appropriately and effectively.

6.3.1 You can delegate the responsibility for a task but not the accountability. This means that, although you can ask someone to carry out a task for you, you could still be held accountable if something goes wrong. You should only delegate or refer to another member of the team if you are confident that they have been trained and are both competent and indemnified to do what you are asking.

6.3.2 If you delegate a task to another member of the team who does not feel that they are trained or competent to carry it out, you must not take advantage of your position by pressuring them into accepting the task.

6.3.3 You should refer patients on if the treatment required is outside your scope of practice or competence. You should be clear about the procedure for doing this.

6.3.4 If you ask a colleague to provide treatment, a dental appliance, or clinical advice for a patient, you should make your request clear and give your colleague all the information they need.

6.3.5 If you need to refer a patient to someone else for treatment, you must explain the referral process to the patient and make sure that it is recorded in their notes.

Standard 6.4 Only accept a referral or delegation if you are trained and competent to carry out the treatment and you believe that what you are being asked to do is appropriate for the patient.

6.4.1 If a colleague asks you to provide treatment, a dental appliance, or clinical advice for a patient, you must ensure that you are clear about what you are being asked to do and that you have the knowledge and skills to do it.

6.4.2 If you do not think that what you have been asked to do is appropriate, you should discuss this with the colleague who asked you to do it. You should only go ahead if you are satisfied that what you have been asked to do is appropriate. If you are not sure, you should seek advice from your professional association or defence organisation.

Standard 6.5 Communicate clearly and effectively with other team members and colleagues in the interests of patients.

6.5.1 You should document any discussions you have with colleagues about a patient's treatment, including any decisions you have reached or changed, in that patient's notes.

Standard 6.6 Demonstrate effective management and leadership skills if you manage a team.

6.6.1 You should make sure that all team members, including those not registered with the GDC, have:

- a proper induction when they first join the team;
- performance management, including regular appraisals;
- opportunities to learn and develop;
- a hygienic and safe working environment;
- a work environment that is not discriminatory;
- opportunities to provide feedback; and
- a way to raise concerns.

6.6.2 You should make sure that relevant team members are appropriately registered with the GDC or another healthcare regulator, appropriately in-training to be registered with the GDC or another healthcare regulator and that those who are registered with the GDC are also indemnified.

6.6.3 You should encourage all team members, including those not registered with the GDC, to follow the guidance in this document, as well as following it yourself.

6.6.4 You should make sure that you communicate regularly with all members of the team and that all members of the team are involved and included as appropriate.

6.6.5 You must encourage, support, and facilitate the continuing professional development (CPD) of your dental team.

6.6.6 Medical emergencies can happen at any time in a dental practice. You must make sure that:

- there are arrangements for at least two people to be available within the working environment to deal with medical emergencies when treatment is planned to take place;
- all members of staff, including those not registered with the GDC, know their role if there is a medical emergency; and
- all members of staff who might be involved in dealing with a medical emergency are trained and prepared to do so at any time, and practise together regularly in a simulated emergency so they know exactly what to do.

6.6.7 You should ensure your team has:

- good leadership;
- clear, shared aims; and
- an understanding of their roles and responsibilities.

6.6.8 You should ensure that all the members of your team understand their roles and responsibilities, including what decisions and actions have, and have not, been delegated to them.

6.6.9 You should discuss all new policies and procedures with your colleagues so that everybody understands them and make sure that all team members are aware of their responsibility to comply with them.

6.6.10 You should display information about the members of your team (including their registration number where appropriate), in an area where it can be easily seen by patients.

6.6.11 You should display the following information in an area where it can be easily seen by patients:

- the fact that you are regulated by the GDC; and
- the nine principles contained in this document.

Principle 7 – Maintain, Develop, and Work within your Professional and Skills

Patient expectation:

- To receive good quality care.
- That all members of the dental team:

- are appropriately trained and qualified;
- keep their skills up to date;
- know their limits and refer patients as appropriate; and
- work within current laws and regulations.

Standard 7.1 Provide good quality care based on current evidence and authoritative guidance.

7.1.1 You must find out about current evidence and best practice which affect your work, premises, equipment, and business, and follow them.

7.1.2 If you deviate from established practice and guidance, you should record the reasons why and be able to justify your decision.

Standard 7.2 Work within your knowledge, skills, professional competence, and abilities.

7.2.1 You must only carry out a task or a type of treatment if you are appropriately trained, competent, confident, and indemnified. Training can take many different forms. You must be sure that you have undertaken training which is appropriate for you and equips you with the appropriate knowledge and skills to perform a task safely.

7.2.2 You should only deliver treatment and care if you are confident that you have had the necessary training and are competent to do so. If you are not confident to provide treatment, you must refer the patient to an appropriately trained colleague.

7.2.3 You must only work within your mental and physical capabilities.

Standard 7.3 Update and develop your professional knowledge and skills throughout your working life.

7.3.1 You must make sure that you know how much continuing professional development (CPD) activity is required for you to maintain your registration and that you carry it out within the required time.

7.3.2 You should take part in activities that maintain, update, or develop your knowledge and skills. Your continuing professional development (CPD) activity should improve your practice. For more information, see the GDC's advice on CPD.

Principle 8 – Raise Concerns if Patients Are at Risk

Patient expectation:

- That the dental team will act promptly to protect their safety if there are concerns about the health, performance, or behaviour of a dental professional or the environment where treatment is provided.
- That a dental professional will raise any concerns about the welfare of vulnerable patients.

Standard 8.1 Always put patients' safety first.

8.1.1 You must raise any concern that patients might be at risk due to:

- the health, behaviour, or professional performance of a colleague;
- any aspect of the environment where treatment is provided; or
- someone asking you to do something that you think conflicts with your duties to put patients interests first and act to protect them.

You must raise a concern even if you are not in a position to control or influence your working environment.

Your duty to raise concerns overrides any personal and professional loyalties or concerns you might have (for example, seeming disloyal or being treated differently by your colleagues or managers).

8.1.2 You must not enter into any contract or agreement with your employer or contracting body which contains a 'gagging clause' that would prevent you from raising concerns about patient safety or restrict what you could say when raising a concern.

Standard 8.2 Act promptly if patients or colleagues are at risk and take measures to protect them.

8.2.1 You must act on concerns promptly. Acting quickly may mean that poor practice is identified and tackled without there being a serious risk to patient safety. If you are not sure whether the issue that worries you amounts to a concern that you should raise, think about what might happen in the short or longer term if you did not mention the issue. If in doubt, you must raise your concern.

8.2.2 You should not have to prove your concern for it to be investigated. If the investigation shows that there was no problem, the fact that you raised the concern should not be held against you as long as you were justified in raising the concern. Remember that you must put patients' interests first and act to protect them. If you fail to do so by not raising a concern, your own registration could be at risk.

8.2.3 Where possible, you should raise concerns first with your employer or manager. However, it may not always be appropriate or possible to raise concerns with them, particularly if they are the source of your concern.

8.2.4 If it is not appropriate to raise your concern with your employer or manager, or if they fail to act on your concern, you must raise your concerns with your local commissioner of health or with the appropriate body from the following:

- the Care Quality Commission;
- Healthcare Inspectorate Wales;
- the Regulation and Quality Improvement Authority;
- Healthcare Improvement Scotland. You can also get advice from your defence organisation or professional association.

8.2.5 If you think that the public and patients need to be protected from a dental professional registered with the GDC, you must refer your concern to us. This may be appropriate when:

- taking action at a local level is not practical; or
- action at a local level has failed; or
- the problem is so severe that the GDC clearly needs to be involved (for example, issues of indecency, violence, dishonesty, serious crime, or illegal practice); or
- there is a genuine fear of victimisation or deliberate concealment; or
- you believe a registrant may not be fit to practise because of his or her health, performance or conduct.

8.2.6 You must refer concerns about other healthcare professionals to the relevant regulator.

Standard 8.3 Make sure if you employ, manage, or lead a team that you encourage and support a culture where staff can raise concerns openly and without fear of reprisal.

8.3.1 You must promote a culture of openness in the workplace so that staff feel able to raise concerns.

8.3.2 You should embed this culture into your policies and procedures, beginning with staff training and induction.

8.3.3 You should encourage all staff, including temporary staff, staff on different sites, and locums, to raise concerns about the safety of patients, including the risks that may be posed by colleagues, premises, equipment, or practice policies.

8.3.4 You must not offer staff contracts which contain a 'gagging clause' that would prevent them from raising concerns about patient safety or restrict what they could say when raising a concern.

Standard 8.4 Make sure if you employ, manage, or lead a team that there is an effective procedure in place for raising concerns, that the procedure is readily available to all staff and that it is followed at all times.

8.4.1 You must make sure there are written procedures in place to enable staff members to raise concerns. This means:

- being aware of and adhering to current laws and regulations;
- supporting staff members who raise concerns;
- taking steps to tackle any shortfalls in the standards and performance of staff; and
- having systems in place for supporting staff who may be having problems with their health, behaviour, or professional performance.

8.4.2 When a member of your team has raised a concern, you must:

- take the concerns seriously;
- maintain confidentiality when appropriate;
- investigate promptly and properly and make an unbiased assessment of the concern;
- keep the staff member who raised the concern advised of progress, explaining any action taken or reasons for not taking action; and
- ensure that you monitor the action you take to solve the problem.

Standard 8.5 Take appropriate action if you have concerns about the possible abuse of children or vulnerable adults.

8.5.1 You must raise any concerns you may have about the possible abuse or neglect of children or vulnerable adults. You must know who to contact for further advice and how to refer concerns to an appropriate authority such as your local social services department.

8.5.2 You must find out about local procedures for the protection of children and vulnerable adults. You must follow these procedures if you suspect that a child or vulnerable adult might be at risk because of abuse or neglect.

Principle 9 – Make Sure your Personal Behaviour Maintains Patients' Confidence in You and the Dental Profession

Patient expectation:

- That all members of the dental team will maintain appropriate personal and professional behaviour.
- That they can trust and have confidence in you as a dental professional.
- That they can trust and have confidence in the dental profession.

Standard 9.1 Ensure that your conduct, both at work and in your personal life, justifies patients' trust in you and the public's trust in the dental profession.

9.1.1 You must treat all team members, other colleagues, and members of the public fairly, with dignity and in line with the law.

9.1.2 You must not make disparaging remarks about another member of the dental team in front of patients. Any concerns you may have about a colleague should be raised through the proper channels.

9.1.3 You should not publish anything that could affect patients' and the public's confidence in you, or the dental profession, in any public media, unless this is done as part of raising a concern. Public media includes social networking sites, blogs, and other social media. In particular, you must not make personal, inaccurate, or derogatory comments about patients or colleagues.

9.1.4 You must maintain appropriate boundaries in the relationships you have with patients. You must not take advantage of your position as a dental professional in your relationships with patients.

Standard 9.2 Protect patients and colleagues from risks posed by your health, conduct or performance.

9.2.1 If you know, or suspect, that patients may be at risk because of your health, behaviour, or professional performance, you must consult a suitably qualified colleague immediately and follow advice on how to put the interests of patients first.

9.2.2 You must not rely on your own assessment of the risk you pose to patients. You should seek occupational health advice or other appropriate advice as soon as possible.

Standard 9.3 Inform the GDC if you are subject to criminal proceedings or a regulatory finding is made against you anywhere in the world.

9.3.1 You must inform the GDC immediately if you are subject to any criminal proceedings anywhere in the world.

9.3.2 You must inform the GDC immediately if you are subject to the fitness to practise procedures of another healthcare regulator, either in the United Kingdom or abroad.

9.3.3 You must inform the GDC immediately if a finding has been made against your registration by another healthcare regulator, either in the United Kingdom or abroad.

9.3.4 You must inform the GDC immediately if you are placed on a barred list held by either the Disclosure and Barring Service or Disclosure Scotland.

Standard 9.4 Cooperate with any relevant formal or informal inquiry and give full and truthful information.

9.4.1 If you receive a letter from the GDC in connection with concerns about your fitness to practise, you must respond fully within the time specified in the letter. You should also seek advice from your indemnity provider or professional association.

9.4.2 You must cooperate with:

- commissioners of health;
- other healthcare regulators;
- hospital trusts carrying out any investigation;
- the Coroner or Procurator Fiscal acting to investigate a death;
- any other regulatory body;
- the Health and Safety Executive; and
- any solicitor, barrister, or advocate representing patients or colleagues.

General Dental Council

The General Dental Council (GDC) is the regulatory body for dentistry. The GDC are there to protect patients by ensuring the public maintain confidence in the profession, and to regulate the dental team.

The GDC follows the Dentist Act 1984 that provides them with the legislation framework which allows them to:

- Grant registrations to professionals who meet the requirements to work as a dental professional in the UK.
- Set standards for the registered professionals and educational sector to abide by at all times.
- Form investigations around any reports of misconduct or fitness to practice.
- Regulate the continuing professional development (CPD) that is required of dental care professionals.

Before 2006, dentists were solely responsible for the care that the patient received in the practice, even though the dental nurse also played a part in the service that was provided. If anything below standard took place, all responsibility was placed onto the dentist. In 2006, the GDC opened the Dental Care Professional Register which all professionals, such as hygienists and therapists working within dentistry had to obtain a registration to work. Dental nurses joined that register in 2008 along with dental technicians. As being a dental nurse is now a profession within its own right, as a registered professional it comes with the responsibility to work within the parameters expected of the profession. This removes the entire responsibility from the dentist and spreads it across the staff within the practice. As a registered professional, you are responsible for your own actions while caring for patients unless it can be proven that your employer knowingly prevented the act of profession from yourself. The GDC produced the Standards for the dental team document to set out the standards of conduct for all dental professionals. It specifies nine principles which set out what patients can expect from their dental professionals, which include dentists, dental nurses, dental hygienists, dental therapists, orthodontic therapists, dental technicians, and clinical dental technicians.

The nine principles that a registered dental professional must follow are the following:

1) Put patients' interests first.
2) Communicate effectively with patients.

3) Obtain valid consents.
4) Maintain and protect patient's information.
5) Have a clear and effective complaints procedure.
6) Work with colleagues in a way that is in patients' best interest.
7) Maintain, develop, and work within your professional knowledge and skills.
8) Raise concerns if patients are at risk.
9) Make sure your personal behaviour maintains patients' confidence in you and the dental profession.

If these standards are not met at any point, then the professional risks being removed from the register and not being able to work within the profession.

While working as a professional, it is understandable that you may want to extend your duties by completing extra courses or post registration courses. This is an excellent way to develop your skills. To gain further understanding of what scope you can work under, the GDC published a document called the Scope of Practice which provides details of additional tasks you can complete under your registration.

Further details of all GDC publications can be found at http://www.gdc-uk.org.

See more in Chapter iv. Roles and responsibilities.

Fitness to Practise

To work as a dental professional in the UK there are requirements that you have to meet. This includes dentists, orthodontists, therapists, hygienists, and dental nurses. If at any point a report is made against a dental professional relating to their conduct or competence within their scope of practice, the GDC will take the necessary steps to protect the patient and ensure that the person in question has adequate training that allows them to complete their role in line with the standards set out. The GDC's responsibility is to mitigate the risk.

The term fit to practise means: the person has the appropriate skills, knowledge, character, and health to practise the profession safely and effectively. The GDC would also investigate acts that the professional had taken that may not directly be linked to the profession, such as criminal acts. Depending on the outcome of the investigation, there are a few outcomes for any case:

- No further action.
- Issue a reprimand.
- Provide conditions onto registration.
- Suspend registration.
- Removal of the individual from the register.

There is also an appeals procedure for anyone going through investigation who doesn't agree with the outcome.

NICE Guidelines

The National Institute for Health and Care Excellence (NICE) provides national guidance on the promotion of good oral health and the prevention and/or treatment for poor oral health in all areas. All NHS contractors in England should comply with all NICE guidelines. Wales, Scotland and Northern Ireland are able to use the NICE guidelines to form their own set of regulations. As an oral health educator, you play a big part in promoting good oral hygiene which complies fully with NICE guidelines.

Clinical Governance

Clinical governance requires a quality assurance system to be put in place for the practice. This ensures a consistent quality of care is provided and that reviews are made frequently to always improve the quality of the service. Areas covered to ensure the safety of a practice's patients are:

- **Infection control:** ensuring the effectiveness of infection control measures in place within the dental practice.
- **Health and safety:** ensuring that all legal obligations towards health and safety are in place and being followed correctly by the practice.
- **Radiation protection:** ensuring that all legal obligations towards radiation are in place and being followed correctly by the practice.
- **GDC compliance:** ensuring the compliance required by the GDC.
- **Risk and incident management:** ensuring that any incidents are reviewed, investigated throughout, and risks are minimised to prevent the same incident happening again.
- **Performance monitoring:** ensuring that all staff are performing to the best of their ability in order to provide the high-quality care and service that is expected of them. If the performance is not up to standard, then action plans are put into place for improvement; this would be completed under regular reviews.

Clinical Audit

A clinical audit is essential for the clinical governance that came into force for NHS dentists in 2001. It was put in place to assess individual dentists and the different aspects of practice. In order for dentists to continue to learn, if there is room for improvement of services then clinical audits will identify these areas so improvements can be implemented. Quality assurance programmes can be delegated to suitably trained staff to carry out the audit. As an oral health educator, you may be involved in some clinical audit procedures, this could involve visits out of the practice to social areas such as schools or care homes. You could be auditing on the number of people you see and how receptive they are to the advice depending on the environment.

Information Governance

Information governance is a system that has been implemented for healthcare, corporate, and information technology (IT) organisations as part of the quality assurance system. It is set out to ensure the safety of the personal and patient information that a dental practice holds. It is closely related to patient confidentiality, general data protection, and freedom of information. The Department of Health set out a toolkit which was originally known as the IG toolkit, now known as the DSP toolkit, to ensure NHS healthcare providers are monitoring their own compliance.

Scope of Practice

The Scope of Practice document was put into place to regulate dental care professionals in their roles and give a full explanation of what they can do under their professional title. For example, in the GDC Scope of Practice it states that all members of the dental team must have regular training in medical emergencies and all members of the team should be able to provide sufficient evidence of this, should it be required.

Under the title 'dental nurse' in the Scope of Practice document, it states the duties the professional is expected to carry out and any additional duties that may be asked of them or they may want to take on board themselves – one of which is oral health educator. As a qualified dental nurse, you have the ability to refer to this document to confirm any duties asked of you or to expand what duties you do have.

General Data Protection Regulations

The General Data Protection Regulation (GDPR) replaces the Data Protection Act 1998. The change will remain in place even after the UK has left the EU.

It gives individuals greater control over their own personal data.

The new GDPR legislation was released 25 May 2018.

GDPR will condense the Data Protection Principles into six areas, which are referred to as the Privacy Principles: They are:

1) Settings must have a lawful reason for collecting personal data and must do it in a fair and transparent way.
2) Settings must only use the data for the reason it is initially obtained.
3) Settings must not collect any more data than necessary.
4) It has to be accurate and there must be mechanisms in place to keep it up to date.
5) Settings cannot keep it longer than needed.
6) Settings must protect the personal data.

These privacy principles are supported by a further principle – accountability. This means that settings must not only do the right thing with data but must also show that all the correct measures are in place to demonstrate how compliance has been achieved. Staff are trained on data protection, and a named data protection officer appointed.

Consent for data collection must be freely given, specific, informed, and unambiguous. It must be specific, clear, prominent, opt-in, properly documented, and easily withdrawn. It must be opt-in and not silent. It must be separate from other terms and conditions. There must be a simple way for people to withdraw their consent.

Individuals have the following rights:

- The right to be informed.
- The right of access.
- The right of rectification.
- The right to erasure.
- The right to restrict processing.
- The right to data portability.

- The right to object.
- The right not to be subject to automated decision-making including profiling.

Access Requests

Patients have the right to request information about the data we hold. As professionals, we can:

- Refuse or charge for requests that are deliberately unfounded or excessive.
- If we refuse, then we must state the reason why.
- Requests must be made in writing to the Practice Manager.

Disclosure Without Patient Consent

- When requested by the Business Services Authority to discuss the patient's claim.
- To assist in identification of a driver or passenger involved in a road traffic accident where facial trauma prevents identification otherwise (under the Road Traffic Act 1988).
- To provide information to a parent or guardian.
- When it is in the public's best interest, e.g. a known criminal.
- When disclosing as part of a court order under the Prevention of Terrorism Act 1989 or under the Police and Criminal Evidence Act 1984.
- When disclosure is necessary to a solicitor or debt agency to enable them to pursue a legal claim against the patient on behalf of the dentist.

Safeguarding

All dental professionals have a responsibility for the wellbeing of their patients, and this can include the protection of children and vulnerable adults. Each practice will have a safeguarding policy and protocol in which all professionals with a safeguarding issue should report.

Several types of abuse may be seen. The Care Act 2014 catagorises different forms of abuse, some of which include:

Neglect – where there is failure to meet the person's basic needs e.g. food, drink, clothing, shelter, lack of medical, and dental treatment. Things to look out for include:

- Malnourishment.
- Failure to comply with professional advice that is in the best interest of the person.
- Inappropriate clothing.
- Persistently dirty, uncared for appearance.
- Untreated illness including dental caries.
- Difficult behaviour e.g. distractive, withdrawn, seeking attention.

Emotional abuse – involves adverse effects on emotional development, e.g. bullying and making them feel unwanted. Signs to look out for include:

- Self-harm.
- Inability to cope with normal life events.
- Becoming agitated and distressed when left alone.
- Drug or alcohol abuse.
- Educational problems.

Sexual abuse – involves the victim being forced to take part in sexual acts of a physical nature or watch graphic material. Signs to look out for include:

- Physical trauma to the lips and oral cavity that is not easily explained.
- Evidence of lesions that may indicate sexually transmitted diseases.
- Inappropriate sexual knowledge beyond the age of the victim.
- Pregnancy in a child or vulnerable adult who is unlikely to be in a relationship.

Physical abuse – hitting, shaking, scalding, burning, biting, etc. Signs to look out for include:

- Bite marks.
- Orofacial trauma, e.g. ears, cheeks, intra-oral soft tissue.,
- Bilateral injuries, e.g. two black eyes instead of one.
- Soft tissue injuries, e.g. scratches, bruises, etc.
- Flinching away at sudden movements or noises.

Mental Capacity

Capacity means that a person must be able to understand, believe, retain, and communicate the information they have been told. If they cannot do any of these things, then their capacity is questioned.

No one else is able to consent to treatment on behalf of a competent adult, and all adults must be assumed to be competent and able to make their own decisions unless they demonstrate otherwise. Incompetent adults are those who, for reasons of mental incapacity or illness, cannot give informed consent to treatment because they do not have the capacity to reach an informed decision on their own behalf. The dentist needs to assess the patient to determine the validity of the consent.

Further information can be found in the Mental Capacity Act 2005.

In summary the following are able to give consent:

- Parent of guardian of a child to the age of 16.
- Gillick-competent child to the age of 16 in England and Wales.
- 16–18 year old of sound mind, in England and Wales.
- 16 year old in Scotland and Northern Ireland.
- Competent adult.
- Dentist on behalf of an incompetent adult, when in the patient's best interests and with an agreeing second opinion from another professional.

Health and Safety

All dental practices are governed by the Health and Safety at Work Act (1974). Among other legislation and in compliance with the HSE (Health and Safety Executive), employers are required to ensure that all employees are kept safe.

Risk assessments should be carried out within the workplace to identify any potential risks. The potential risk and its prevention through controls is then fully set out to ensure that the employee undertaking the duties is fully aware of the health and safety risks of any task.

The following has to be considered when carrying out a risk assessment:

1) Identify the hazard (procedure or chemical, etc.).
2) Identify who may be harmed.
3) Evaluate the risk.
4) Control the risk.
5) Record the risk assessment findings.
6) Review the assessment process.

The GDC asks for fitness to practise requirements from all dental care professionals:

- Always undergo and follow training provided when using materials and equipment.
- Follow all practice policies in relation to health, safety, and welfare issues.
- Never misuse any materials or equipment on the premises – in particular materials or equipment that are specifically meant to reduce or eliminate hazardous risks.
- Never enter certain hazardous areas without authorisation to do so.
- Always report any failures in equipment or procedures to senior member of staff.
- Always report any suspected health problem that will affect their normal work to a senior member of staff.

General Safety

To prevent hazards:

- Correct storage, handling, and use of drugs – to be locked in a cabinet.
- Good ventilation and a scavenging system for nitrous oxide during inhalation sedation.
- Follow manufacturer's instructions.
- Wear PPE.
- Non-slip flooring and unobstructed entries and exits.
- No dust traps in clinical areas.
- Guards around fires/heaters to prevent burns.
- No sharp edges on furniture.
- No trailing electrical cables.
- PAT testing carried out and written records kept.
- All electrical equipment disconnected overnight to help prevent fires.
- Fully stocked first aid kit.

Revision

Revision 1: Acronyms and Abbreviations

Acronyms and abbreviations are a good way to help you remember some of the very important information required.

Table R1.1   Table of abbreviations.

ABCDE	Airway, Breathing, Circulation, Disability, Exposure
ANUG	Acute Necrotising Ulcerative Gingivitis
BDA	British Dental Association
BDS	Bachelor of Dental Surgery
BLS	Basic Life Support
BNF	British National Formulary
BPE	Basic Periodontal Examination
BSA	Business Services Agency
CCG	Clinical Commissioning Group
CDT	Clinical Dental Technician
COSHH	Control of Substance Hazardous to Health
CPD	Continuing Professional Development
CPITN	Community Periodontal Index of Treatment Needs
CPR	Cardiopulmonary Resuscitation
CQC	Care Quality Commission
DBS	Disclosure and Barring Service
DCP	Dental Care Professional
DMF	Decayed, Missing, Filled (in secondary teeth) (dmf in primary teeth)
DRSABC	Danger, Response, Shout, Airway, Breathing, Circulation
DSE	Display Screen Equipment
DUWL	Dental Unit Water Lines
DSP	Data Security and Protection
eCPD	Enhanced Continuing Professional Development

(Continued)

Questions and Answers in Oral Health Education, First Edition. Chloe Foxhall and Anna Lown.
© 2021 John Wiley & Sons Ltd. Published 2021 by John Wiley & Sons Ltd.
Companion website: www.wiley.com/go/foxhall/oral-health-education

Table R1.1 (Continued)

EMQ	Extended Matching Questions
FAST	Face, Arms, Speech weakness, Time to call 999
FDI	Fédération Dentaire Internationale/World Dental Federation
GDC	General Dental Council
GDP	General Dental Practitioner
GDPR	General Data Protection Regulations
HIS	Healthcare Improvement Scotland
HIW	Healthcare Inspectorate Wales
HSCA	Health and Social Care Act
HSE	Health and Safety Executive
HTM 01-05	Health Technical Memorandum 01-05 (decontamination)
HTM 04-01	Health Technical Memorandum 04-01 (legionella prevention)
HTM 07-01	Health Technical Memorandum 07-01 (management of healthcare waste)
ICO	Information Commissioner's Office
ILS	Intermediate Life Support
INR	International Normalised Ratio
IOTN	Index of Orthodontic Treatment Need
LSAB	Local Safeguarding Adult Board
LSCB	Local Safeguarding Children Board
MCA	Mental Capacity Act
MCQ	Multiple Choice Questions
MHRA	Medicines and Healthcare products Regulatory Agency
MMR	Measles, Mumps, and Rubella
NCSCT	National Centre for Smoking Cessation and Training
NEBDN	National Examining Board for Dental Nurses
NHS	National Health Service
NICE	National Institute for Clinical Excellence and Health
NME	Non-Milk Extrinsic sugar
NSAID	Non-Steroidal Anti-Inflammatory Drugs
NUG	Necrotising Ulcerative Gingivitis
OHA	Occupational Health Advisor
OHE	Oral Health Educator
OHI	Oral Health Instructions
PCO	Primary Care Organisation
PCT	Primary Care Trust
PDP	Personal Development Plan
PDU	Preventative Dental Unit
pH	Measure of Acidity and Alkalinity

Table R1.1 (Continued)

PPE	Personal Protective Equipment
PPM	Parts Per Million
QA	Quality Assurance
RIDDOR	Reporting of Injuries, Diseases, and Dangerous Occurrence Regulations
ROC	Record of Competence
SCC	Squamous Cell Carcinoma
SMART	Specific, Measurable, Attainable, Realistic, Time-based objectives
SWOT	Strength, Weakness, Opportunities, and Threats (analysis)
UNC	University of North Carolina (periodontal probe)
WHO	World Health Organisation

Revision 2: Methods of Retaining Information

Revision is something that is personal to you and everyone successfully revises in different ways. Some ways of revision that work well for you may not work as well for a classmate. This chapter is to give you some useful tips for revision, aside from using this book. You can complete these with a class member or by yourself.

1) 'Mind map'

   A mind map is usually focused around a topic; for example, if you were revising plaque you would write plaque in the middle of your page. It doesn't matter what size paper you complete this on, but it is suggested that to get the best out of your mind map you use paper no smaller than A4. With your subject in the centre of the page, you can circle that and then from that you can create branches going towards the outside of the page; these can labelled with subtitles which can also be branched off again with facts or any other information about that topic. A mind map is also known as a spider diagram, the centre topic being the spider's body and the branches acting as the legs. You can also add colour to these to create connections between different topics.

2) Revision cards

   Revision cards can be a great way to revise and test yourself on current knowledge. You can buy packs of revision cards from most stationary shops; however, you can also make your own. You can start cutting a piece of A4 paper or card into six equal sized rectangles, write the question onto one side and the full answer on the reverse. You can use revision cards by giving them to someone to test your knowledge and then mark down the answers you got incorrect, revise those areas, and then try again. It is also good to shuffle the cards once you have completed them, so you don't get into a habit of remembering the answers in a certain order.

3) Group work

   Working alongside other class members can be a great way to learn and revise. Everyone has different strengths and weaknesses while learning; one of your weaknesses could be the strength of the person who is sitting next to you. You can learn a lot from other people, so you should embrace this where you can. Even if you cannot physically meet up with other students, you could talk over the phone or online to gain help from each other.

Questions and Answers in Oral Health Education, First Edition. Chloe Foxhall and Anna Lown.
© 2021 John Wiley & Sons Ltd. Published 2021 by John Wiley & Sons Ltd.
Companion website: www.wiley.com/go/foxhall/oral-health-education

4) Recordings

Recording yourself and replaying it is an extremely useful way of revising. For example, when you put some headphones in and listen to a song, after a few times playing it on repeat you begin to sing along with the song. This works the same way with revision; if you record yourself talking through a topic and then listen to it while completing another activity, you may find that your next test on this topic produces higher scores.

5) Practical work

Practical work can be a beneficial way of revising. When working in a dental practice, you will often be completing some of the tasks expected of you as an oral health educator without realising it. For example, your practice manager asks you to create a new post-operative instructions leaflet for a patient with an orthodontic appliance; this information would be typed up and then you can apply this to your revision.

6) Scenarios

Ask a colleague to pose as a patient during an oral health education session; they can act as a patient would, asking questions while you guide them through the session with help from your lesson plan. You can provide information and then you can receive some constructive criticism on how to improve or if you missed anything.

7) Visual posters

If you have a clear work or revision space, you may want to display some images or diagrams that you create from your class work. Displaying images and diagrams around you can subconsciously help you revise; as you are looking at them without realising it, you take in that information, and if asked a question based on this subject, you can imagine the diagram to help you answer it.

There are many other ways to revise, such as re-writing or typing your class work to help you take in what you are reading, reading and speaking to colleagues, which will all provide you with useful information. Remember to try and change the way you revise so you can learn what helps you and what doesn't. Revision is unique and there will be a way that is best suited to you.

Revision 3: Caries

Dental caries is a progressive bacterial disease that damages calcified areas of the tooth.

It will only occur after eruption. It is a common disease found in populations having a high refined sugar diet.

For caries to occur there must be three things present:

1) an erupted tooth
2) refined carbohydrates (sugar)
3) bacterial plaque.

It also takes TIME for a cavity to form.

Aetiology

The word 'aetiology' is mainly used in medicine, and it simply means the cause behind something; e.g. caries will form when refined carbohydrate and bacterial plaque is present.

Early stages of plaque 'acquired pellicle' become invaded with bacteria.

Sugars diffuse through the plaque and they are broken down and an acid is produced as a by-product.

Bacterial Plaque

The bacteria present for caries to occur are:

- Acidogenic group – these produce acid and remove mineral salts – **Streptococcus mutans** and **Lactobacillus.**
- Proteolytic group – these dissolve proteins – **Clostridia.**

The acidogenic group removes mineral salts first. When the caries reaches the dentine, the proteolytic group begins to act by dissolving proteins.

Questions and Answers in Oral Health Education, First Edition. Chloe Foxhall and Anna Lown.
© 2021 John Wiley & Sons Ltd. Published 2021 by John Wiley & Sons Ltd.
Companion website: www.wiley.com/go/foxhall/oral-health-education

Facts:

- The pH balance of the mouth is approximately 6.8.
- When we consume foods/drinks containing sugar they diffuse through plaque and are broken down.
- Acid is produced as a by-product; this action is immediate.
- The calcium and phosphate ions are withdrawn from the tooth when the pH level falls below 5.5. This process is called demineralisation, or more commonly known as acid attack.
- It can take from 30 minutes to 2 hours for the pH to reach a safe level (above 5.5). This is when the calcium and phosphates are replaced back into the tooth from the saliva. This process is called remineralisation.
- Saliva helps to neutralise and wash away the acid. Cheese can also help neutralise the acid in the mouth as it has a chemical reaction with saliva.
- The process of demineralisation and remineralisation is called the ionic seesaw.

Stephan's Curve

The Stephan's curve is a great way to measure and show the cariogenic challenge to a tooth. The critical pH value varies between individuals. The cariogenic challenge (cariogenicity) is measured as the area delimited by the critical pH and the Stephan's curve shown shaded in the diagram.

Cariogenic means producing caries, usually due to diet.

The Stephan's curve shows the demineralisation and remineralisation process after meals.

The pH level will drop to critical in less than 2 minutes at each sugar intake and will take from 30 minutes to 2 hours to rise back to a safe level.

Frequent sugar intake will allow the pH to remain at a critical level for longer periods, which is when caries occurs.

It is acceptable to consume sugary items three times per day at mealtimes. There is then adequate time for remineralisation to take place.

The Process of Caries

- The early lesion
  This is generally first seen as an opaque white spot on the surface of enamel. The spot becomes rough and can become stained if present for a while. This stage is much easier to see on smooth surfaces than fissures.
  This is the cause of unsightly white or brown boxes seen after orthodontic brackets have been removed following poor oral hygiene.
  If the lesion progresses, the surface of the enamel disintegrates and a minute cavity forms.
- The open cavity
  Once the caries has reached the dentine, it spreads more rapidly than in the enamel. The enamel edges become undermined and the supporting enamel breaks off to form a progressively larger cavity.

The tooth may be symptomless but can still become sensitive to hot, cold, and sweet things. If the caries reaches the pulp, the pain becomes much worse and longer lasting.
- Periapical abscess

When a tooth dies, the necrotic (dead) contents of the pulp canal causes an infection around the apex of the tooth. There are two types of periapical abscess:

1) Acute periapical abscess: the tooth is very sore to touch with swelling and the patient may have a slight fever.
2) Chronic periapical abscess: the tooth may or may not be sore to touch and has an apical radiolucency on the radiograph. The pus may break through the bone and form a discharging sinus.

A periapical abscess always arises from a dead tooth as opposed to a periodontal abscess, which is usually associated with a vital (living) tooth.

Caries Distribution in the Mouth

Caries can start from stagnation areas and attack some teeth more than others. The molars are the most commonly involved, followed by the premolars and the upper incisors. The lower incisors and canines are the teeth least likely to be affected.

Main Stagnation Areas

- fissures
- occlusal pits
- interproximal surfaces near the contact point
- the buccal surfaces near the gingival margin
- displaced teeth
- partially erupted teeth
- dentures or orthodontic appliances
- poor margins on fillings and crowns.

Root Caries

Carious lesions are termed either primary (new lesions on previously unrestored surfaces) or secondary (new caries around existing restorations). They occur on the crowns of teeth and exposed root surfaces. Root caries lesions are seen in patients with gingival recession which can be as a result of periodontal disease or abrasion.

Root caries can attack the dentine directly, which is exposed due to gingival recession. This forms an open cavity.

Root caries is a widespread problem in adults and appears to be increasing. This is perhaps because more and more adults are retaining their own teeth into old age. Also, investigation and treatment of periodontal disease exposes the root surface, making the root more susceptible to bacterial attack.

Risk factors associated with the high prevalence of root caries among older adults include:

- chronic medical conditions
- xerostomia (decreased salivary flow)
- radiation treatment

- physical limitations
- diminished manual dexterity, e.g. arthritis or Parkinson's disease
- Alzheimer's disease or dementia
- diabetes
- changes in dietary habits.

One or more of these risk factors or life changes, which are more common among older adults, can increase root caries in an individual who has not had dental caries for many years.

Working as an oral health educator, you are working to advise patients on how to maintain a good oral health standard and prevent caries.

Revision 4: Fluoride

There are three ways in which fluoride works:

1) Systemically – affects the teeth during formation. This is ingested/swallowed.
2) Topically – acts as an enzyme inhibitor, reducing acid production from sugar by plaque. This coats the teeth.
3) Assists the plaque and saliva to remineralise the enamel.

Enamel is made up of crystals. The most common constituents are calcium and phosphate in the form of hydroxyapatite crystals. Fluoride alters the structure of these crystals. Ion exchange then takes place and hydroxyapatite is then converted into fluorapatite. Fluorapatite is more resistant to acid attacks than hydroxyapatite.

All oral health educators should recommend fluoride to help prevent caries.

Calcium absorbs fluoride; therefore, fluoride should not be given with milk or milk products as it will counteract the effect of the fluoride.

Fluoride occurs naturally in some water, fish, tea and many other food stuffs.

Forms of Fluoride

If there is little or no fluoride in the water supply, then it is advisable to have supplements to help strengthen teeth. The following dosage is recommended for people living in areas with less than 0.3 ppm in the water supply. Manufacturer's instructions must always be followed when using supplements (Table R4.1).

For people living in areas where the water has 0.3–0.7 ppm of fluoride, then the recommended dosage should be halved.

Questions and Answers in Oral Health Education, First Edition. Chloe Foxhall and Anna Lown.
© 2021 John Wiley & Sons Ltd. Published 2021 by John Wiley & Sons Ltd.
Companion website: www.wiley.com/go/foxhall/oral-health-education

Table R4.1 Table of dosage levels
of fluoride for children.

Age	Dose (mgF)
6 mo to 3 yr	0.25
3 to 6 yr	0.50
6 yr and over	1.00

Drops and Tablets

These are available in different milligrams for different age groups. These are only available on prescription from a dentist.

Advantages

- Easy to administer to young children.
- Gives a systemic and topical effect.
- Inexpensive.
- Suitable for children who have difficulties with mental or physical health.
- Free on prescription.
- Long shelf life.
- Lactose-free tablets available.

Disadvantages

- Can often be a low priority within the family.
- Parents often forget.
- Parents need to be very motivated.
- It is easy to squeeze the bottle rather than measure the drops properly.
- Requires a long-term commitment.
- Parents don't like to give children tablets.

Fluoride Mouth Rinses

Fluoride mouth rinses are not available on prescription, but can be purchased from a chemist or supermarket.

Rinsing should be carried out for 1–2 minutes and at a different time to brushing, therefore giving the teeth an extra topical coating (e.g. at lunch time)

Young children can swallow the rinse; therefore, it is not recommended for children under the age of 8. This is predominantly to prevent fluorosis.

Fluoride Toothpaste

Fluoride toothpaste became widely available in the 1970s.

There are 3 concentrations

- 400–600 ppm
- 1000 ppm
- 1500 ppm.

The concentration of fluoride can be found on the box of the toothpaste.

For children aged 0–3 years, a smear of toothpaste should be used, containing at least 1000 ppm fluoride.

For children aged 3–6 years, a pea sized amount of toothpaste should be used, containing 1350–1500 ppm fluoride.

This is subject to change based on the child's oral health risk.

Parents have to be careful how much toothpaste they are putting on the brush, only a pea size amount is needed.

Fluoridated Salt

Administration of fluoride via salt intake is an alternative where the local situation is not suitable for water fluoridation. Studies have produced consistent data indicating its effectiveness in reducing caries. The production of fluoridated salt for a particular country of geographical area should be centralised with strong technical support to ensure controlled production. This works in the same way as fluoridated water in helping to reduce caries. The amount added will help protect against caries without causing any harm to anyone using it. It is recommended by the World Health Organisation for communities where water fluoridation is not possible. Concentration of fluoride in salt must be based on studies of salt intake and the availability of fluoride from other sources. The fluoride concentration should appear on the salt packaging.

Nearly 200 million people worldwide consume fluoridated salt to help protect their teeth against caries. It is available in Europe, Central and South America, and the Caribbean.

Fluoridated Milk

Fluoridated milk is milk in one of its various forms, e.g. fresh, powdered, or UHT, to which a small amount of fluoride has been added to protect against caries.

Over 672 000 children drink fluoridated milk at school; 40 000 of these are in Britain.

Fluoridated milk has been used as a fluoride source, especially for young children through school programmes. A number of studies have shown it to be effective. However, it has had limited exposure as a public health measure. In primary schools and nurseries in England, the usual amount added to a carton of milk is 0.5 mg fluoride.

Gels and Varnishes

Gels are used in the dental surgery, not the home. They are applied to the teeth in trays, which can be uncomfortable for children. Varnishes are applied directly to the tooth, normally by use of an applicator.

Overdose

If a child takes an overdose of fluoride, then take the following steps:

- Find out how much has been taken.
- Inform the dentist or local hospital if there is no dentist available.
- Get the child to drink as much milk as possible (this may cause the child to be sick).
- Attend the hospital.
- Write up all records.

The National Fluoride Information Centre (NFIC) is an online source of independent fluoride information. It offers advice and resources for health professionals and the public on all types of fluoride use and delivery.

Fluoridation

Fluoridation is the addition of fluoride in the public water supply. Many substances are added to our water supplies before the water comes out of the tap. Adding fluoride is the same.

Worldwide, hundreds of water works already add fluoride to the water. There are even several in this country, so the system is now routine and well tested.

One of only two chemicals is used for fluoridation. These are added as a liquid to the water supplies at the water treatment works.

The chemicals are delivered to the water works and held in large storage tanks. Fluoride is then fed into the smaller tanks designed to hold only enough for a day's supply. From these smaller tanks, fluoride is pumped into the mains water at the correct level. Pumps run at full capacity so, if a breakdown occurs, smaller not greater amounts of fluoride will be passed into the water supply. At all stages, strict regulations mean the chance of an accident is extremely low, especially as the tanks only hold enough fluoride for one days supply.

The British Fluoridation Society was founded in 1969 by a group of concerned professionals anxious to see an improvement in the dental health of the UK population by the implementation of government policy for water fluoridation. Founder members include Eric Lubbock MP. The society has always been a multi-disciplinary organisation, and has enjoyed the support of politicians from all political parties.

Fluoride in water acts systemically and topically.

Fluoride occurs naturally in some water. Hartlepool in Newcastle is naturally fluoridated, whereas fluoride is artificially added to water in Birmingham.

Fluoride is at the optimum level when it is at, or above, one part of fluoride to every million parts of water; 1 ppm ($1\,\mathrm{mgl}^{-1}$) is the recommended level.

Fluoridation is reported to reduce caries by at least 45%.

Epidemiological studies have been carried out comparing fluoridated areas to non-fluoridated areas. The results show there is a greater reduction in caries in fluoridated areas.

Water fluoridation reduces the number of decayed, missing, and filled teeth by on average just over two teeth per child. Water fluoridation increases the percentage of children totally free from caries by approximately 15%.

The reduction in the number of decayed, missing, or filled teeth following fluoridation is greatest in those areas with the highest levels of caries at the beginning. Copies of the DMF league tables can be found on the fluoridation society website or from your local public health offices.

The University of York NHS Centre has reviewed the evidence of the dental benefits of water fluoridation for reviews and dissemination. The York Review included 26 studies representing the best available evidence on the effectiveness of water fluoridation.

Advantages of Water Fluoridation

- Inexpensive.
- Most effective method.
- Reaches all of the population.
- Reduces dental caries in all of the population.
- Controlled.

Disadvantages of Water Fluoridation

- Mass medication.
- If fluoride toothpaste is also used and swallowed, mild fluorosis may occur.
- Who pays for it?

York Review

The York Review was commissioned by the Chief Medical Officer of the Department of Health and involved 'an up to date expert scientific review of fluoride and health'. The University of York published it in September 2000.

Water fluoridation has been designated one of the ten most important public health measures currently available (Achievements in Public Health 1900–1999: Fluoridation of drinking water to prevent dental caries. Reported by Division of Oral Health, National Centre for Chronic Disease Prevention and Health Promotion, CDC: Centres for Disease Control and Prevention), and this publication was a milestone in its continuing and developing evaluation. The British Fluoridation Society also regularly introduces new schemes to continue and develop education.

The York Review was a timely reminder of the need to maintain and update the research database supporting all public health measures.

Mrs Catherine McColl vs Strathclyde Regional Council

Judgement given on 29 June 1983

On 13 September 1978, Strathclyde Regional Council as a statutory water authority agreed to cooperate with local Health Boards by fluoridating water supplies for which they were responsible. In October 1979, an elderly citizen of Glasgow (Mrs Catherine McColl) applied for an interdict to restrain Strathclyde Regional Council from implementing its decision. This was allowed pending court hearings.

Legal aid was granted to Mrs McColl. In brief, Mrs McColl's submission was that fluoridation is unsafe, ineffective, and illegal.

Lord Jauncey was appointed to judge the hearings: expert witnesses were alerted and invited to give written and verbal evidence to the court. The hearings, held in the Court of Session, Edinburgh, commenced on 23 September 1980 and continued until 26 July 1982. The court sat for 201 days making it the longest and costliest case in Scottish legal history. The judges took almost 12 months to consider the massive evidence and gave his verdict at 10 am on 29 June 1983.

The verdict was that there was no evidence to suggest that fluoride at the proposed concentration would have an adverse effect upon health. Lord Jauncey also upheld the effectiveness of water fluoridation and found that 'fluoridation of water supplies in Strathclyde would be likely to reduce considerably the incidence of caries'.

Knox Report

In 1980, the Department of Health and Social Security commissioned a Working Party with the remit of assessing all published evidence on the alleged linkage between human cancer and fluoridation.

Members of the Working Party were authorities in epidemiology, cancer research, pathology, statistics, and water treatment. The Working Party published its 116-page report on 14 January 1985.

Professor Knox and his team concluded in the report that 'We have found nothing in any of the major classes of epidemiological evidence which could lead us to conclude that either fluoride occurring naturally in water on fluoride added to the water supply is capable of causing cancer.'

Revision 5: Visual Aids

A visual aid is something that is used in a lesson that students can see to help them learn. It can range from a tooth model to a poster.

Types of Visual Aids

- a worksheet
- a photograph
- post
- leaflet
- story picture
- food packets
- toothbrush
- a tooth
- tooth model
- a video
- a jigsaw.

The most important aspect is that the aid used is relevant to your teaching subject. Good use of a visual aid is the difference between a boring lesson and an interesting and enjoyable one.

Advantages of Visual Aids

- Help the student learn.
- Can make the lesson more interesting.
- Students remember what they have seen more than what they have heard sometimes.
- If teaching on a one-to-one basis, then it gives the student something to look at other than the educator.
- Helps to make the student alert.

Questions and Answers in Oral Health Education, First Edition. Chloe Foxhall and Anna Lown.
© 2021 John Wiley & Sons Ltd. Published 2021 by John Wiley & Sons Ltd.
Companion website: www.wiley.com/go/foxhall/oral-health-education

Disadvantages of Visual Aids

- Can be expensive.
- Homemade visual aids can look a bit tatty,
- May not be able to see the aid if seated at the back of the room.
- The visual aid could get broken.
- Leaflets and posters produced by manufactures are often advertising something.

Computers

The computer is an excellent resource. There are many programs that can be used for designing leaflets and posters.

The internet is an excellent resource. Most companies, dental hospitals, and dental associates have their own websites with valuable, useful information.

Leaflets

Leaflets produced by companies are often advertising something which can often take the attention of the reader away from the actual message. Leaflets can be used during a teaching session to highlight the points that have been discussed. They can also be placed in strategic areas, e.g. waiting rooms, for patients to pick up and read or take away.

Assessing Literature

Patients often forget what they have been told in the surgery for a number of reasons. Therefore, if you give the patient a leaflet to take away, you should ensure it is appropriate for that patient.

Ease of Reading Index (ERI)

- readability
- jargon
- layout
- range of topics covered
- interest.

Readability

There are a number of tests available which determine the reading age of the literature. It is important not to give a child a leaflet that is above their reading age. Remember that children learn to read lower case first.

Jargon

Jargon is profession-specific language that other people may not understand. For example, in dental terminology – gingiva or periodontal disease. The patient may know it as gum disease.

Ensure that dental terms used are easily understood; the less jargon used the better.

Layout

If the leaflet has too much writing on it, it gives the appearance of being boring. Too many pictures can be confusing. Coloured print on coloured backgrounds can be difficult to read. Graphs and charts can confuse the reader.

Range of Topics Covered

If too many topics are covered then it can confuse the reader. If there is one topic you wish the patient to read, then a leaflet with lots of topics can detract from the main one.

Interest

If the reader is interested, then they will enjoy the literature. It is up to you to stimulate that interest.

Ethnic Issues

In today's multicultural society, it would be a good idea to have your leaflets translated into different languages to give to those who may have English as a second language. The Health Development Agency stocks a good range.

Aims

An aim is a guide to a teacher.

It consists of one, two, or three sentences explaining what you want the students/patients to be able to do. It is a general statement.

An aim is not measurable!

Example

During the session, the students will develop a better understanding of hidden sugars in foods and drinks.

Here is a list of words often used in writing aims:

- further understanding of
- improve knowledge
- improve ability
- increase knowledge
- appreciate
- know.

Examples

- improve their knowledge of the causes of tooth decay;
- gain a greater understanding of the causes of gum disease;
- improve knowledge on effective toothbrushing;
- know about sugar in foods.

Objectives

An objective is what the student/patients will be able to do at the end of the session. It is a doing word, so the recipient will be able to 'do' something by the end of the session or lesson. An objective describes terminal behaviour. An objective is measurable by time.

Objectives should always begin with:
'By the end of the session, the students/patients will be able to . . .'

If it states: 'the patient will be able to do . . .' then it is not measurable as you haven't said when they will be able to do it by.

To ensure you have achieved any objectives you have set, you must give the students/patients the tasks stated in your objectives.

Examples

- Identify – you would ask the patient during the lesson to identify, e.g. food.
- List – during or at the end of the session, you would ask the student/patient to compose a list of, e.g. food.
- Describe – during or at the end of the session, you would ask the students to describe, e.g. causes of gum disease.

An example list of objectives

- draw
- identify
- state
- demonstrate
- construct
- list
- describe
- pick out
- select
- name
- differentiate
- solve
- make
- recite.

All objectives must be SMART

- Specific
- Measurable
- Attainable
- Relevant
- Time related.

Lesson Preparation

It is important to plan a lesson beforehand.

General Planning

To do this, it is best to complete a lesson plan. This should tell you:

- what you are teaching
- when
- how
- where
- how many
- aims
- objectives
- teaching methods.

A lesson should have:

1) A beginning – giving a brief introduction of who you are and what you expect the students/patients to learn during the session (your objectives).
2) A middle – where you give the new information.
3) An end (conclusion) – rounding up the lesson. If you have not already tested your objectives, then you should do so in this section.

Background Information

Before beginning to complete a lesson plan, you should consider the following background information:

- How many students/patients will there be?
- Will everyone fit in the room?
- Do the students/patient share a previous knowledge of the subject?
- What facilities are available?
- Are there any electrical points?
- Is there a TV or computer available?
- The time available to you.
- Do the students have any learning disabilities?

- How old are the group?
- What are their ethnic groups?
- What are their social backgrounds?

Teaching Methods

It is important to use a range of teaching methods. You should choose your teaching methods carefully, giving thought to whom you are teaching and their age.

Lecture/talk – This is one person talking to the group over a set period of time.

Discussion – This is where the tutor will begin a discussion with the group. The tutor must be in control to ensure the group stays on the topic of the discussion.

Diary – Students/patients keep a personal diary of their own. It can be on their personal development during a set period of study or on a set topic, e.g. a diet sheet.

Role play – The learners take on roles, e.g. children can act out a visit to the dentist.

Demonstration – This is where the teacher demonstrates a certain action.

Practical – This is where the student is performing the practical task. A practical task should not take up the whole lesson.

Project/assignment – This is where the student would carry out information searching, a literature study, data treatment /analysis, material compilation, and then final reporting.

Game – This is an ideal teaching method for children, e.g. putting an unsafe sugary snack into the correct box.

Evaluation

Evaluation is the process by which the effects and effectiveness of teaching can be determined.

One of the first models to evaluate healthcare quality was developed by Donabedian and included the elements of: structure, process, and outcomes.

For example, dental hygiene and quality assurance:

1) **Structure** – the resources needed to perform the task; in this case, the physical facilities, equipment, records and management, and support processes which enable the dental hygienist to practice.
2) **Process** – the act of doing the task; in this case, the procedures and activities undertaken by the dental hygienist.
3) **Outcome** – the results; in this case, of dental hygiene care.

There are many different types of assessment that be split up into the following groups:

- written
- oral
- practical
- aural.

It is important to assess your teaching to ensure you have achieved your objectives.

Written Assessments

This is where the student/patient is involved in writing a:

- test
- essay
- questionnaire
- examination.

Oral – This is where the tutor asks questions. It can be during or after the session. It can also take the form of an oral examination.

Practical/observation – You can assess a practical session/lesson by watching the student/patient at the time of the lesson, e.g. by observing a toothbrushing session.

Aural – This is a useful type of assessment when learning a foreign language, e.g. listening to a foreign language and answering a question in that same language.

Revision 6: Muscles of Mastication

Figure R6.1: Table of the muscles of mastication and their functions.

Muscle name	Point of origin	Point of insertion	Action
Temporalis	Temporal bone in the cranium	Coronoid process of the mandible, passing under the zygomatic arch	Pulls the mandible backwards and closed
Masseter	Outer surface of the zygomatic arch	Outer surface of the mandibular ramus and angle	Closes the mandible
Lateral pterygoid	Lateral pterygoid plate at the base of the cranium	Outer surface of the mandibular ramus and angle	Contracting the mandible towards to bite the anterior teeth edge to edge and pulls the mandible to the side
Medial pterygoid	Medial pterygoid plate at the base of the cranium	Inner surface of mandibular ramus and angle	Closes the mandible

All four of these muscles receive nerve impulses from the fifth cranial nerve, the trigeminal nerve; these nerve impulses are what form the contraction of the muscle allowing us to move our jaw.

Questions and Answers in Oral Health Education, First Edition. Chloe Foxhall and Anna Lown.
© 2021 John Wiley & Sons Ltd. Published 2021 by John Wiley & Sons Ltd.
Companion website: www.wiley.com/go/foxhall/oral-health-education

Revision 7: Oral Conditions

Oral conditions can form on any patient and are not always serious or life threatening; however, during a routine appointment the soft tissues should always be checked. As an oral health educator, it is important for you to understand oral conditions and what causes them.

Candidiasis

- Thrush

  This is a fungal infection generally characterised by white patches and ulceration on the tongue and other oral mucosal surfaces, which can be wiped off with gauze. It is caused by infection with the microorganism *Candida albicans*. It is an infection but can be treated with antifungal preparations such as a mouthwash or lozenge. If thrush is left untreated, it can lead to angular cheilitis.

- Angular cheilitis

  This is characterised by redness, cracking of radiating fissures from the corners of the mouth (where the top and bottom lip meet). It is sometimes covered with a white membrane, which can be wiped off. It normally accompanies intra-oral candidiasis. It should be treated the same as thrush except cream can be applied externally, but the intra-oral candidiasis should also be treated. It is usually seen in older people.

- Denture stomatitis

  Stomatitis means a sore or inflammation inside the mouth. Not cleaning dentures properly can lead to infections and inflammation. A denture left in the mouth overnight can cause thrush infections. It may start as a red patch on the palate. Though patients may complain it is uncomfortable, it is not generally sore. If left untreated, it will become sore. It is essential in the management of denture stomatitis that patients remove their dentures at night and clean them thoroughly. The infection will be treated the same as thrush. Some cases are associated with poor diet, anaemia, diabetes, or Human Immunodeficiency Virus/Acquired Immune Deficiency Syndrome (HIV/AIDS).

Questions and Answers in Oral Health Education, First Edition. Chloe Foxhall and Anna Lown.
© 2021 John Wiley & Sons Ltd. Published 2021 by John Wiley & Sons Ltd.
Companion website: www.wiley.com/go/foxhall/oral-health-education

Other Conditions

- Denture soreness

  The denture wearer may suffer with an area of ulceration/irritation if the dentures fit poorly and irritate the gingiva. The management of this problem is for the denture wearer to leave the denture out of the mouth until the ulcer has healed. A chlorhexidine mouthwash can help the discomfort and can aid healing. The denture should then be adjusted by the dentist.

- Xerostomia

  This is more common in older patients. It is a direct result of age, due to a reduction in the flow of saliva. People suffering with xerostomia can experience difficulty with eating and speech. Artificial saliva preparations can be used. Fluoride mouth rinses can also be beneficial. Remember: saliva helps to neutralise acid; so the less saliva, the more at risk of caries the patient will be.

  Dry mouth can be caused by radiation treatment to the head and neck, damage to salivary glands or by certain drugs; antispasmodics, tricyclic antidepressants, some antipsychotic drugs, and highly active antiretroviral therapy (HAART) drugs used by people living with HIV.

  There are many artificial saliva products including sprays and lozenges that the dentist can prescribe which can help ease the symptoms. The reduced saliva flow can increase the chance of caries. It is important to brush with a fluoride toothpaste and keep sugary foods and drinks to mealtimes only.

- Ulcers (aphthous ulcers)

  Ulcers can occur singularly or in crops. They are found on the inside of the lips and cheeks or on the tongue. They can take from between 1 or 2 weeks to heal depending on their aetiology. They fall into three groups:

  - Major aphthous ulceration – large ulcers usually greater than 5mm in diameter occurring singularly or in small numbers
  - Minor aphthous ulceration – 2–5 mm in diameter occurring in crops around the mouth
  - Herpetiform Aphthous ulceration – not related to a primary herpetic infection but similar in appearance with similar small ulcers.

    The main feature of ulceration is that the aetiology is unknown and that they are recurrent.

    Treatment should include investigation which may include blood tests to eliminate systemic causes.

- Halitosis

  Halitosis is the clinicial name for bad breath. This can be a difficult and embarrassing problem to deal with. Good oral hygiene should be recommended with the use of interdental cleaning and mouthwash. A scale and polish may also be required by the dentist or hygienist. If this treatment doesn't cure the halitosis, then further examinations will be needed.

- Herpes (cold sore)

  This is a common form of ulceration. It is a viral infection. It can produce small crops of grey ulcers and there is usually a tingling or burning sensation before the ulcer appears. Herpes labialis virus remains dormant in the trigeminal ganglion.

Cold sores are caused by the herpes simplex virus. A first cold sore usually occurs in childhood. The virus infects through the moist 'inner' skin that lines the mouth. It is commonly passed on by skin contact, such as kissing.

After the first infection, the virus settles in a nearby nerve sheath and remains there for the rest of your life. For most of the time, the virus lies dormant (inactive) and causes no symptoms. However, in some people the virus becomes 'active' from time to time. When activated, the virus multiplies and travels down the nerve sheath to cause cold sore blisters around the mouth. Some people have cold sores often; others only now and then. Some things that may trigger the virus to activate and cause a cold sore include:

- Sunshine – strong, direct sunlight may trigger cold sores in some people.
- Stress – or just being 'run down' for whatever reason.
- Illness – cold sores may occur during feverish illness such as colds, coughs, and flu.
- Menstruation – cold sores are common around the time of monthly periods.

Symptoms of cold sores

- Tingle or itch.
- Normally around lips or nose.
- After the tingle, the blister usually appears.
- The blisters can weep.
- The blister can then become a scab.
- The scab will disappear slowly leaving no scar.

Infectious

- Passed on from skin-to-skin contact, e.g. kissing.
- Avoid kissing a newborn baby if a cold sore is present.

Treatments

- If sunlight triggers the cold sore, then use a sunscreen lip balm.
- Soothing gel or cream as prescribed by a pharmacist.
- Painkillers if required.

Antiviral creams are used for the treatment of cold sores. They do not kill the virus, but prevent it from multiplying. They have little effect on existing blisters, but may prevent them from getting worse.

- Bruxism
  Bruxism is commonly known as tooth grinding. This is the clenching together of the upper and lower jaw accompanied by the grinding of the upper and lower teeth.

It affects between 10% and 50% of the population depending on the particular study.

Bruxism is a subconscious behaviour so many people do not realise that they are doing it! Often it is the partner who tells them about the night time sounds that the bruxism produces.

Although it can occur during waking hours, bruxism most frequently occurs while we sleep. During sleep, the biting force can be up to six times greater than the pressure during waking hours. Consequently, significant damage is much more likely to occur with this nighttime bruxism.

Oral Malignancy (Squamous Cell Carcinoma)

Although the aetiology of oral cancer is complex, epidemiological studies have implicated tobacco smoking and drinking alcohol as the major causes of the disease in Westernised countries. Separately, the factors increase the risk of oral cancer; but combined, this risk multiplies.

Tobacco

In Scotland, the main risk factor for oral cancer is cigarette smoking. Stopping smoking causes a sharp decline in risk of oral and pharyngeal cancer with, after 10 years, no increase in risk comparative to non-smokers. Pipe smoking also leads to an increased incidence of the disease. In some population groups, oral cancer also shows a strong association with chewing tobacco. Combinations of tobacco betel nuts are responsible for high regional cancer rates worldwide.

Alcohol

Increased risk of oral and pharyngeal cancer has been linked with heavy consumption of spirits, wine, and beer. It is thought to promote carcinogenesis by a number of mechanisms; e.g. alcohol increases the effects of topical carcinogens, such as those found in tobacco.

In addition, long-term misusers of alcohol often have nutritional deficiencies, which may affect the normal maturation process of the oral mucosa. Many modern mouthwashes sold for oral hygiene purposes contain alcohol in significant concentration. It is best to recommend an alcohol-free mouthwash to help with the prevention of oral cancer, although it is not yet established how the oral mucosa reacts to the preparations in the long term.

Sunlight

Ultraviolet light is important in the aetiology of lip cancer, due to actinic radiation damage. It is more common in outdoor workers, people who live in sunny climates, and people who holiday in hot/sunny places. Sunlight is not important in the development of lip cancers inside the mouth.

Nutritional Aspects

Nutritional deficiencies (in particular iron) produce atrophy of the oral mucosa and may allow ingress of various carcinogenic substances. It is well known that diets high in antioxidant vitamins (A, C, and E) appear to offer protection against the development of oral cancer. To reduce the risk of oral cancer, it would be a good idea to advise a diet high in fruit and vegetables.

Infective Causes

Evidence suggests that there are strong links between Human papilloma viruses (HPV) and some types of mouth and throat cancers. Potentially malignant lesions, e.g. chronic hyperplastic candidosis of the oral mucosa, showing evidence of candida infection, have a higher risk of malignant transformation.

Oncogenes

Disturbance to the regulation of cell growth and cell death can result in neoplasia. Genes in normal cells (proto-oncogenes) code for proteins involved in the regulation of cell growth and differentiation; abnormalities in these genes (oncogenes) or their expression, may be involved in the development of cancer generally. The role of cancer promoting genes (oncogenes) and tumour suppressor genes in relation to oral cancer is a complex and rapidly developing field.

Signs

While the majority of oral cancers apparently arise in normal mucosa, some oral carcinomas are preceded by pre-malignant changes.

- White patches and red patches of the oral mucosa should be biopsied to demonstrate the presence or abscess of pre-malignant changes.
- Identification of such changes gives warning of risk, and presents an opportunity for close follow-up and the provision of preventative measures.
- Although white patches (leukoplakia) of the oral mucosa are more common, red patches (erythroplakia), and white patches with a red component (speckled leukoplakia), should be viewed with greater suspicion.
- These lesions have much higher potential than leukoplakia for malignant transformation.
- Some of these lesions are already squamous cell carcinomas, or carcinomas in situ, or show severe epithelial dysplasia
- Chronic trauma to the oral mucosa, e.g. a sharp tooth, may promote neoplastic change. The removal of sources of chronic irritation should be routine practice in the dental surgery. Thereafter, an altered mucosa should be reviewed within one month.
- Look for any non-healing lumps or ulcers, warty lumps, nodules, or thickening of the oral mucosa. Again, if the mucosal abnormality persists, assessment by an expert should be undertaken with a view to mucosal biopsy.
- Oral lichen planus is thought by some to be a pre-malignant lesion in around 1% of patients. The erosive and plaque-like forms may be more prone to malignant transformation.
- Neck swellings and changes in speech are late signs of oral cancer.

Other Factors

Although oral cancer occurs in all layers of society, social deprivation is identified as a specific risk factor for the disease. Of growing concern are the patients with no obvious risk factors such as smoking and alcohol. These patients are often young and have aggressive tumours with poor prognosis.

Dry mouth can be caused by radiation treatment to the head and neck, damage to the salivary glands, or by certain drugs. There are many artificial saliva products, sprays, and lozenges that a dentist can prescribe. Reduced saliva flow can increase the risk of caries. It is important to brush with a fluoride toothpaste and keep sugary foods and drinks to mealtimes only. External or internal radiation therapy can often cause damage to the salivary glands, leading to a permanently dry mouth. Due to lack of saliva, there is more risk of dental caries, so it is particularly important to have regular dental check-ups. Some cancer patients find that chemotherapy causes a sore throat, difficulty swallowing, and in some cases partial or complete loss of taste.

If patients are going to have a course of chemotherapy, they must visit the dentist as soon as possible to make sure any dental treatment is finished before they start. Chemotherapy can cause gum ulcers or gums to bleed. Regular appointments with the dental hygienist should help to keep this under control. The hygienist will also check the patient is brushing correctly and will check that they are maintaining a good oral hygiene routine at home.

Acquired Immunodeficiency Syndrome

HIV stands for the Human Immuno-deficiency Virus. This is a virus that people can become infected with and that they can then pass on to other people.

When someone becomes infected with HIV, it begins to attack their immune system, which is the body's defence against illness. This process is not visible.

A person infected with HIV may look and feel well for many years and they may not know they are infected. Then the person's immune system weakens and they become vulnerable to illnesses, many of which they would normally fight off.

When a person is infected with HIV, they are likely as time goes by to become ill more and more often. A person is said to have AIDS when, usually several years after first becoming infected with HIV, they have developed one of a number of particularly severe illnesses.

HIV is present in the sexual fluids and blood of infected people. It can also be in the breastmilk of infected women. It is also possible for an infected woman to pass on the virus to her unborn baby either before or during birth. Contact with any person's blood is risky if it allows the virus to pass into another person's body through cuts or grazes in their skin. This is why it can be risky to have a needle stick injury.

It is **not** normally possible to become infected with HIV through:

- insect/animal bites
- sharing cutlery and crockery
- touching, hugging or shaking hands
- eating food prepared by someone with HIV.

There is currently no cure for AIDS, although in many countries greatly improved medical treatments are now available. These are not a cure, but can stop people from becoming ill for many years. The treatment consists of drugs that have to be taken every day for the rest of someone's life.

HIV is a virus and, like other viruses, when it is in a cell in the body it produces new copies of itself. With these new copies, HIV can go ahead and infect other previously healthy cells. It is easy for HIV to spread quickly through the billions of cells in the body if it is not stopped from reproducing itself. Antiretroviral treatment for HIV infections consists of drugs which work against HIV infection itself, by slowing down the reproduction of HIV in the body. The drugs often used are:

- anti-HIV drugs
- antiretroviral
- HIV antiviral drugs.

AIDS and the Oral Cavity

The oral cavity often shows signs of this disease. It manifests itself in the following ways:

Fungal Infections

- angular cheilitis
- thrush.

Viral Infections

- Herpes – painful ulcers found on the lips; can be treated with acyclovir cream.
- Hairy leukoplakia – usually found in the lateral border of the tongue. It appears white with red cracking radiating fissures. Can be treated with acyclovir preparations.

Periodontal Infections

- HIV positive people are more susceptible to gingivitis.
- HIV related gingivitis causes redness and swelling of the gingiva, loss of interdental papilla and sometimes ulcers and bleeding or pain. If this is untreated, it may rapidly progress to HIV-related periodontitis (known as necrotising ulcerative periodontitis or NUP), or inflammation around the teeth. Soft tissue may be destroyed and the underlying bone exposed, and the bone itself can be destroyed, loosening the teeth and causing severe pain. NUP resulting from HIV needs to be seen by a dentist experienced in HIV care.
- Gingival erythema – red band on the gingival margin with spontaneous gingival bleeding.
- Acute necrotising ulcerative gingivitis.

Other Gingival Diseases

Neoplasia

- Non-Hodgkin's lymphoma – rapidly growing swelling occurring anywhere in the mouth.
- Karposi's sarcoma – red, purple, blue nodule normally found on the palate.

Miscellaneous lesions

- ulceration
- necrotising stomatitis
- salivary gland disease.

Revision 8: Oral Hygiene Aids

Toothpaste

Fluoride toothpaste became widely available to the UK in the early 1970s. Because of the use of fluoride within toothpaste, there has been a decrease in caries prevalence.

Fluoride toothpaste is recommended and should be used; however, care should be taken with the strength of fluoride for young children due to fluoridation and fluoride supplements.

There are three strengths of fluoride toothpaste available over the counter:

- 400–600 ppm
- 1000 ppm
- 1300–1500 ppm.

PPM stands for parts per million and is the measurement used when looking at fluoride strength.

The British Dental Association has an accreditation scheme, which is awarded to tooth-pastes that satisfies certain criteria.

The amount of toothpaste that is used depends on age. A child under 3 should only use a smear of toothpaste and then anyone over 3 should use a pea size amount. Once brushing is complete, the excess should be spat out but not rinsed out as this reduces the topical effect of the fluoride.

When children are using toothpaste, they should be supervised to ensure they are not swallowing excessive amounts as this can become harmful to a child.

Normal Toothpaste

A toothpaste that is described as 'everyday toothpaste' with 12-hour antibacterial activity holds the following active ingredients:

- Sodium fluoride 0.32% w/w, 1450 ppmF, 0.3% Triclosan, 2.0% Copolymer

The indication is a reduction of dental caries, improvement to gingival health, and reduction in the progression of periodontitis

This type of toothpaste is recommended for all adult patients and patients over the age of 6.

The main claim for this toothpaste is that it has 12-hour antibacterial protection.

Questions and Answers in Oral Health Education, First Edition. Chloe Foxhall and Anna Lown.
© 2021 John Wiley & Sons Ltd. Published 2021 by John Wiley & Sons Ltd.
Companion website: www.wiley.com/go/foxhall/oral-health-education

Sensitive Toothpaste

A sensitive toothpaste contains ingredients to help block exposed tubules, therefore relieving sensitivity. It will contain an ingredient like strontium acetate hemihydrate.

The description for a sensitive toothpaste is an everyday toothpaste for sensitivity relief. The active ingredients are:

- Sodium monofluorophosphate 1.14% w/w, (1500 ppmF), potassium citrate 5.53% w/w

The indication is for relief and protection from dentine hypersensitivity.

This type of toothpaste is recommended for all adult patients with hypersensitivity and patients over the age of 6.

The main claim is unbeatable sensitivity relief and overall protection.

High Fluoride Toothpaste

This contains more fluoride than an average toothpaste. Recommended for high caries risk patients and those who require extra protection, such as: adults with exposed caries present, highly cariogrenic diet or medication, reduced saliva flow; orthodontic appliance wearers, and senior patients, etc.

The product description is an everyday high fluoride toothpaste. The ingredients are:

- Active sodium fluoride 0.019% w/w (2800 ppmF)

The indication is treatment and prevention of dental caries. It should be used for patients over the age of 10.

- Active sodium fluoride 1.1% DPF.

The indication is treatment and prevention of dental caries. It should be used for patients over the age of 16 with a high caries risk, present or potential root caries, xerostomia, orthodontic appliances, overdentures and those with high cariogenic diet or medication.

High fluoride toothpaste contains one of the highest fluoride concentrations currently available in the UK. It is clinically proven to reduce caries.

Whitening Toothpaste

This contains ingredients that break down and remove stains, therefore restoring the teeth to their natural colour. It will contain an ingredient like triclosan.

Copolymers are added with the triclosan to help it remain on the teeth longer for a greater effect.

Ingredients in Toothpaste

Abrasives

- approximately 33%;
- these are cleaning and polishing agents, e.g. sodium, silica, metaphosphate, calcium carbonate.

Detergent

- approximately 1–2%;
- this makes the paste foam, e.g. sodium lauryl sulphate.

Binding agent

- approximately 1–5%;
- this prevents the separation of the solid and the liquid ingredients, e.g. alginates, xanthan gums.

Humectants

- approximately 10–30%;
- this retains moisture to prevent the toothpaste from going hard, e.g. glycerol, propylene glycerol.

Flavouring, colour, sweetener

- approximately 1–5%;
- ingredients such as saccharin for a sweetener.

Preservatives

- approximately 0.05–0.5%;
- added to prevent growth of microorganisms, e.g. alcohol, benzoates.

Fluoride

- up to 0.32% or up to 1500 ppm.

Or Monofluorophosphate

- up to 1.14% or up to 1500 ppm.

Interdental Cleaning

Dental Floss

It is important to clean in between teeth daily because this is a front-line of defence in preventing periodontal disease and halitosis.

It allows you to get to the areas beyond the reach of your toothbrush. Using dental floss daily is one of the common ways to clean between your teeth. It is quite common for gums to bleed when you start flossing. It may be a sign that you have some form of gum disease. After a few days of flossing, the bleeding should stop as your gums become healthier.

Patients must always be shown how to use floss:

- The floss should be wound around the second finger of each hand leaving approximately 6 cm in the middle.
- The floss is pulled tight and inserted between the teeth using a back and forward motion.
- The floss is then curved into a C shape against one of the teeth and gently scraped up and down against the tooth to remove plaque subgingivally.

There are different types of floss available:

- waxed
- unwaxed
- tape
- ribbon
- super floss
- ultra floss
- g floss for implants
- floss holder
- flossettes
- flavoured floss.

Interdental Brushes

Interdental brushes are small single tufted brushes that are inserted interdentally to clean interproximal surfaces and the gingival crevis.

Interdental Wood Sticks

These are designed to clean between the teeth, but care needs to be taken not to damage the gingiva. These are for people who require an alternative to floss.

They are triangular in shape and made of wood. They are used to clean between the teeth and along the gum line. It is necessary to moisten the stick with water or saliva, and then insert it between the teeth with the flat edge next to the gum line. Use a gentle in and out motion to clean plaque from between the teeth. Also run the tip gently along the gum line to remove additional plaque. A new wood stick should be used for each cleaning session.

Disclosing Agents

These colour the plaque on teeth to make it easier to see and therefore easier to clean off. Disclosing agents are available in tablet or liquid form. They are made from harmless vegetable dyes called erythrosin.

Anti-Plaque Mouth Rinses

The dentist or hygienist would normally suggest the use of these.

Chlorhexidine is the most widely used. It helps to inhibit the production of plaque bacteria, although tooth brushing is still required. Chlorhexidine is available as a rinse and a gel, which can be brushed onto the teeth and gums.

One disadvantage of chlorhexidine is that it causes staining; therefore, it must only be used for a period of a month at a time.

Triclosan, the phenol derivative, has been found to be quite effective when combined with other ingredients, without the disadvantage of staining.

Tongue Scrapers and Cleaning

If you can see any off-colour areas at the back (base) of your tongue, you've found a bad breath breeding ground!

Bacteria live and thrive on the back of our tongues, and the only way to remove as much of this debris as possible is with a tongue scraper or cleaner. Tongue scraping twice a day when brushing is more effective at eliminating halitosis than brushing alone and can actually increase taste sensitivity.

Tongue scrapers or cleaners, which are U shaped devices made from plastic or stainless steel, have been around for years but are just recently gaining in popularity. They should be rinsed in hot water after every use. It is even more beneficial to store them in a glass of antibacterial rinse.

Studies suggest that tongue cleaning should accompany brushing and flossing in order to achieve a truly cleansed mouth. Tongue cleaning removes most bacteria and other debris that are the primary source of halitosis and calculus.

Tongue cleaning is comfortable, easy and takes less time than using a rinse. It is a chemical-free process and actually removes plaque and other debris from your tongue, instead of masking it. It is impossible to remove all the bacteria from the mouth as even after a professional scale and polish, bacteria will swarm back.

Revision 9: Plaque

Plaque is composed of bacteria and is a sticky polysaccharide matrix. It is made up of 70% microorganisms and 30% interbacterial substances. It is colourless, which therefore makes it difficult to see.

Plaque sticks to certain areas of the teeth, particularly where tongue, cheeks, and lips can't disturb it.

Plaque forms from saliva, as a thin film. This is called an **acquired pellicle** or **salivary pellicle**. It forms within a short period of time. Approximately 3–8 hours later, the salivary pellicle becomes invaded with gram-positive cocci (bacteria – streptococcus).

About 24 hours after first forming, a small layer of plaque can be seen. Gram-negative bacteria can now be found within the plaque.

Three days after first forming, **spirochaete** and **fusiform** bacteria can now be found.

Seven days after forming, there are fewer cocci bacteria (gram-positive) and more spirochaete and fusiform (gram-negative).

- Subgingival plaque – below the gingival margin. This contains a lot of bacteria and is a soft sticky film
- Supragingival plaque – above the gingival margin. This can often be removed with a toothbrush alone

Gram-Negative/Gram-Positive

Bacteria are difficult to see and identify. One the most important staining methods is the grams method. This uses grams stain and divides bacteria into two groups:

Gram – positive = blue stain

Gram – negative = red stain

Plaque is common in both periodontal disease and caries but there is little evidence to support the theory that 'if plaque is brushed away from our teeth, they will not

Questions and Answers in Oral Health Education, First Edition. Chloe Foxhall and Anna Lown.
© 2021 John Wiley & Sons Ltd. Published 2021 by John Wiley & Sons Ltd.
Companion website: www.wiley.com/go/foxhall/oral-health-education

decay'. Brushing plaque away from the teeth and gums only helps to prevent dental caries and periodontal disease.

A diet high in sugar content often produces accumulations of plaque.

Calculus

If plaque remains on the teeth for any length of time, it can harden and calcify to form calculus/tartar. There are two forms:

- **Subgingival calculus** – forms at and below the gingival margin. Frequently dark brown or green in colour due to the inclusion of haem a product of the breakdown of blood. It is difficult to remove and should only be removed during professional cleaning.
- **Supragingival calculus** – forms at and above the gingival margin. Initially yellow in colour but can quickly become stained by elements of the diet and smoking. Clearly visible and much easier to remove during a professional clean.

Staining

The food and drink we consume can stain supragingival plaque and calculus, e.g. tea, coffee, and Corsodyl mouthwash. The correct term for this staining is extrinsic staining. There are two main types of tooth stain: extrinsic staining on the surface of the tooth and intrinsic staining within the structure of the tooth.

Extrinsic Staining

Extrinsic staining can be caused by:

- Foods and drinks such as tea, coffee, red wine, curry, and berries.
- Poor oral hygiene – plaque can become quite yellow in colour.
- Some antibiotics, e.g. tetracycline.
- Iron tablets can leave clack marks on the teeth.
- Mouthwashes containing the antibacterial chlorhexidine.
- Smoking and tobacco products

Intrinsic Staining

Intrinsic staining can be caused by:

- Fluoride in toothpastes and fluoride drops – causing brown and white flecks (fluorosis).
- Older people can develop brown staining as their enamel wears thin.
- The use of tetracycline antibiotics in children developing teeth (aged 3–12) can cause horizontal brown and grey striping of the enamel surfaces.
- Excessive Fluoride in toothpastes and fluoride drops – causing brown and white flecks (fluorosis)
- trauma – Amelogenesis imperfecta

Periodontal Disease

The main cause of periodontal disease is not brushing teeth and gums effectively. There are also some risk increasing factors:

- smoking
- pregnancy
- anaemia
- leukaemia
- diabetes
- bad diet
- medications.

There are a number of contributing factors to periodontal disease:

- crooked teeth
- dentures
- overhangs on existing fillings
- appliances
- calculus.

There are different types and stages of periodontal disease. The gram-negative stain is present in periodontal disease.

Gingivitis

Bacteria that cause gingivitis are present within plaque. After 7–14 days of the plaque being left on the teeth and gums, the bacteria penetrate the tissues causing inflammation. The body increases the blood flow to the inflamed area to try and fight off the bacteria with antibodies and white blood cells. Because of the increased blood flow, the gums now appear red in colour and are swollen. Bad breath may also be a symptom, although the patient may not be aware of this. The swelling of the gum can cause what is called a false pocket. This pocket harbours more food debris and plaque and the inflammation continues. Toxic enzymes present are collagenase and streptokinase. If the teeth and gums are brushed they will bleed, but bacteria will be removed and the gums will become healthy again in a short time (prevention).

It is better to motivate patients to clean at this stage before the disease progresses.

BPE

BPE stands for Basic Periodontal Examination. The teeth are divided into six quadrants. A Community Periodontal Index of Treatment Needs (CPITN) or World Health Organisation probe (WHO) probe Com is used to determine the presence or absence of:

- bleeding
- calculus
- defective margins of restorations
- pathological pockets.

A probe which has a ball end 0.5 mm in diameter is normally used (CPITN probe).

A colour-coded area on the probe extends from 3.5 to 5.5 mm.

The BPE requires that the periodontal tissue should be examined with a periodontal probe.

BPE Codes

0 = Health Periodontal tissues with no bleeding or pocketing detected.
1 = Bleeding on probing, no pockets above 3.5 mm in depth. No calculus or overhangs present.
2 = Plaque retentive factors present, no pocketing above 3.5 mm in depth.
3 = Pockets present up to 5.5 mm in depth.
4 = Pockets above 5.5 mm in depth.

A newer version of the World Health Organisation (WHO) probe has a second dark band, running from 8.5 to 11.5 mm, to assist in estimating the depth of very deep pockets.

The tip of the probe is gently inserted into the gingival pocket and the depth of insertion is read against the colour coding.

Chronic Periodontitis

This replaces the term 'adult' periodontitis. It describes the most commonly presenting form of periodontitis. It may be localised, affecting just some of the teeth of tooth sites, or more generalised. The term chronic periodontitis does not imply that the condition is resistant to treatment.

When gingivitis reaches the epithelial attachment (fibres), then it becomes periodontitis and this is irreversible.

Gradually, the disease destroys the periodontal membrane and the bone supporting the teeth. A pocket will then form, and this is called a **true pocket.**

This pocket allows more build up of food debris and plaque and this can lead to an abscess forming, known as a **periodontal abscess.**

A periodontal abscess normally appears as a localised painful swelling on the gingiva next to the tooth associated with the deep pocketing.

The abscess usually drains through the pocket.

Periodontitis can be stopped from spreading further, but the damage cannot be reversed.

The teeth eventually become loose and can drift. The root of the tooth can be seen and the teeth will be more sensitive to sensations. You will normally see a layer of calculus and gingival recession.

The patient will suffer from halitosis and may even complain of having a bad taste in the mouth.

Rapidly Progressive Periodontitis

This causes much greater destruction of the supporting structures than would be expected for the age of the patient. There is deep pocketing in relatively young individuals between the ages of 25–35 years.

There is no particular pattern for bone loss. During the active phases, the lesions are acutely inflamed and bleed a lot. There is a higher occurrence in people with systemic disorders.

Aggressive Periodontitis

These forms of periodontitis represent highly aggressive forms of the disease with extensive destruction of the tooth-supporting apparatus. These forms of the disease were previously known as 'early onset periodontitis' and encompass conditions formally known as 'localised juvenile periodontitis' and 'rapidly progressive periodontitis'.
Two forms of aggressive periodontitis are described:

- localised
- generalised.

They cause rapid bone loss, usually around the permanent incisors and the first permanent molars. They are not always associated with poor oral hygiene.
There is seldom any pain associated with this condition.

Necrotising Periodontal Disease

This includes:

- necrotising ulcerative gingivitis;
- necrotising ulcerative periodontitis.

Necrotising Ulcerative Gingivitis (NUG)

Necrotising Ulcerative Gingivitis (NUG) is also known as Vincent's disease. Ulcerative gingivitis was common in the First World War, when it was also known as trench mouth.
The onset of this condition is sudden. It presents the same gum conditions as chronic gingivitis except there are painful ulcers, which can spread. Signs and symptoms of NUG are very easy to spot and include:

- painful gums
- bleeding gums with pressure
- red gums
- crater-like ulcers
- halitosis
- bad taste in mouth.

It tends to occur between the ages of 16 and 30 years old.
There is a distinctive odour associated with this condition and patients complain of an unpleasant or metallic taste in the mouth. The bacteria present are:

- spirochaete
- fusiform.

NUG is thought to be brought on by the following factors:

- smoking
- stress
- poor oral hygiene.

Ulcerative gingivitis responds to penicillin combined with metronidazole. Because toothbrushing is very painful during an attack, the mouth should be kept clean by the use of regular mouthwashes e.g. Chlorhexidine.

The patient should be told to pay careful attention to oral hygiene after the attack in order to help prevent reoccurrence.

Treating NUG requires professional intervention in the form of antibiotics and sometimes dental surgery. Professional cleaning of the gums is also necessary, as is irrigation of the mouth using a saltwater rinse or peroxide solution, as these can often help relieve symptoms. The patient should also:

- rest
- avoid smoking
- avoid eating hot and spicy foods
- have a balanced diet.

Revision 10: Sugars

There are three sugar groups:

- non-milk extrinsic (NME) (also referred to as free sugar)
- intrinsic
- milk sugars.

Within these three groups are many sugars. They can come under many different names, and can be found on the ingredients list of food/drink packaging:

- sucrose
- maltose
- glucose
- dextrose
- fructose
- mannose
- lactose
- honey
- syrup
- glucose syrup.

Quite often, the higher the sugar on the ingredients list, the more of that sugar the product contains.

In order to understand the different types of sugars, the COMA panel (Committee on Medical Aspects) introduced a classification: NME, intrinsic and milk sugars.

Non-Milk Extrinsic

Also referred to as free sugars, these are the sugars found in:

- cakes
- biscuits
- chocolate, etc.

Questions and Answers in Oral Health Education, First Edition. Chloe Foxhall and Anna Lown.
© 2021 John Wiley & Sons Ltd. Published 2021 by John Wiley & Sons Ltd.
Companion website: www.wiley.com/go/foxhall/oral-health-education

This sugar does not occur naturally in the product but is added to it. It is harmful to teeth and can cause caries (cariogenic).

The sugars in this group include:

- sucrose – the main one
- fructose
- glucose.

Intrinsic Sugars

These sugars are found in whole uncooked fruit and vegetables. This sugar is part of the cells found in the food. It does not cause caries as it is broken down and digested in the stomach.

The sugars found in this group are:

- glucose
- fructose
- sucrose.

If the sugar is taken out of the food then this alters the cell structure, this means the sugar will be digested in the mouth, not the stomach, which will cause caries. These sugars will no longer be intrinsic but will be NME sugars.

Milk Sugars

These sugars are found naturally in milk and milk products. This sugar occurs naturally in milk. It does not cause caries as it is digested in the stomach.

Once again, if the sugar is withdrawn from the milk it then becomes cariogenic (causes caries).

The sugar found in this group is:

- lactose.

Sugars can be difficult to understand. It will be helpful to read *The Scientific Basis of Oral Health Education* (by Ronnie Levine and Catherine Stillman-Lowe) as it explains the process of sugars and digestion of sugars.

Artificial Sweeteners

It is important to remember that sugar-free sweets do not cause caries, but they still encourage a sweet tooth so therefore should not be recommended or only eaten at mealtimes. Alternative snacks should be advised for eating between meals, e.g. carrot sticks or crackers.

There are two different categories of sweeteners:

- bulk
- intense.

Bulk

Here is a list of some bulk sweeteners that are available:

- mannitol
- sorbitol
- lactitol
- hydrogenated glucose syrup
- xylitol
- isomalt
- maltitol.

Bulk sweeteners are mainly used to add sweetness to confectionary products. Although artificial sweeteners appear to be non-cariogenic, some do have a mild laxative effect (sorbitol, mannitol).

Intense

Intense sweeteners include:

- aspartame
- acesulfame k
- cyclamate
- neohesperidine dc
- saccharin
- steviol glycosides
- sucralose.

Sugar-free Chewing Gum

Chewing gum increases saliva flow, thereby helping to neutralise plaque acidity. Chewing gum can be beneficial if it is chewed straight after eating as the pH level of saliva returns to normal a lot faster.

Xylitol used in chewing gum has been proven to reduce the growth of acidogenic bacteria in plaque.

Chewing gum can also be beneficial for other medical conditions, e.g. xerostomia.

Sugar-Free Medicines

Artificial sweeteners are now used in some medicines. Sugar-free medicines are becoming more widely available.

A 1989 report from COMA recommended that the government sought means to reduce the use of sugar in liquid medicines. This is within the power of the prescribing doctor in most cases.

The Scottish Executive has also published a report by the National Pharmaceutical Advisory Committee which advises that sugar-free medicines should be used wherever possible.

Prevention of Caries

- Restricting the intake of acidic foods and drinks to mealtimes only.
- Regular use of fluoride, e.g. topical fluoride application, toothpaste, and mouthwash.
- Use of a straw may reduce erosion of front teeth.

Diet Sheets

In order to give dietary advice, you need to know what the patient is eating/drinking throughout the day. One way this can be done is by using a diet sheet.

You will need the patient to complete the diet sheet over a three-day period (one day to be a weekend day) e.g. Thursday, Friday, and Saturday or Sunday, Monday, and Tuesday.

Diet sheets must also include any medicines that are not sugar free.

Advantages of a diet sheet

- You can easily pick out the frequency of sugars.
- The information is written down for you to see easily.
- It makes the patient realise how much between meal sugars they are consuming.

Disadvantages of diet sheets

- Can take a long time to fill in.
- The patient may not be truthful.
- Can the patient read and write?
- The patient may feel intimidated by completing the diet sheet.

Assessment of a Diet Sheet

Diet sheets can be used to assess how many sugar intakes are being consumed during an average day. Here is one way in which you can assess diet sheets.

The chart below shows an example; remember this is sugar intakes, not food intakes.

Day	Meals	In-between	Total
1	3	2	5
2	2	3	5
3	2	1	5
Average:	2	2	4

Day: you must complete it over 3-day period.

Meals: this is the number of meals which contained sugar during the day. Add up all the numbers then divide by 3 (the number of days) $3+2+2=7$ $7\div3=2$ rem. 1/3

In-between: this is the number of snacks/drinks consumed containing sugar. Add up all the numbers then divide by 3 (number of days) $2+3+1=6$ $6\div3=2$

Total: add up all the numbers then divide the total by 3 (number of days). This will then give you the average number of sugar intakes per day $5+5+3=13$ $13\div3=4$ rem. 3

The above person is having an average of 4 sugar intakes – you would advise them to try to bring this down to 3 times per day.

Revision 11: Toothbrushing Techniques

Scrub

The brush is placed perpendicular to the tooth surface at the gum margin. Short horizontal movements are made on the tooth and gum. This technique requires little manual dexterity and is ideal for children.

Instruction should be given to start on the labial and buccal surfaces, then moving onto the palatal and lingual surfaces, and then finishing with the occlusal surfaces.

Starkey

This technique is for an adult brushing a child's teeth.

The child stands in front of the adult and rests their head on the adult's stomach. The adult remains behind the child to support the mandible and uses the scrub technique on the child. This method is easy to use and the adult is able to see into the mouth for erupting teeth or any other problems.

Roll

Place the brush apically nearly parallel to the tooth. Roll the wrist to cover the tooth surface from soft to hard tissues. Scrub the occlusal surfaces. This method does not clean the gingival crevice.

Bass

Angle the toothbrush at 45° apically to the gingival crevice. Press and move the brush back and forth in a short movement. Clean the occlusal surfaces.

This method removes plaque from the cervical and gingival crevices but not from the smooth surfaces. It is an easy method to learn but only a small area is covered at one time.

Questions and Answers in Oral Health Education, First Edition. Chloe Foxhall and Anna Lown.
© 2021 John Wiley & Sons Ltd. Published 2021 by John Wiley & Sons Ltd.
Companion website: www.wiley.com/go/foxhall/oral-health-education

Stillmans

The toothbrush is placed vertically on the gum. Vibrate the toothbrush as in the bass method. Then roll the toothbrush from soft to hard tissues as in the roll method. This technique tends to miss the sulcus area.

Fones

Brush in a circular motion, while teeth are in occlusion. Brush horizontally on lingual surfaces. The interproximal areas do not get cleaned with this method and it can cause damage to the gum.

Charters

Angle the toothbrush at 45° half on the tooth and half on the gum. Make circular motions with the bristle ends remaining stationary. This cleans interproximally but ignores the sulcus and the smooth surfaces.

1

Oral Health Messages

1 A nursing mother has attended the dental practice for oral hygiene advice; which of the following pieces of advice would you not recommend?
   A Clean teeth and gums twice daily with a fluoride toothpaste
   B Don't give a baby sugary drinks
   C For the baby to use a dummy, dip the dummy in jam
   D Start cleaning the baby's teeth as soon as they erupt
   E Use sugar-free medicines

2 The four key oral health messages were put in place for dental health education. When seeing a patient for an educational session, you should provide information from one message per session. Today, you are focusing on the message 'reduce the consumption of sugar and the frequency of intake of food and drink containing sugar'. Which of the following pieces of information is not included in either of the four oral health messages?
   A Raw vegetables are a good alternative to sugary snacks
   B Remove all plaque
   C Sugar should only be consumed three times a day, ideally at mealtimes
   D The prescription and timings of the dental radiographs
   E The appropriate use of fluoride

3 Oral health messages are provided by many people; it should be imperative that the messages given are all the same to stop confusion. Who out of the following would not provide and support oral health messages?
   A Dentists
   B Doctors
   C Midwife
   D Pharmacists
   E Police

Questions and Answers in Oral Health Education, First Edition. Chloe Foxhall and Anna Lown.
© 2021 John Wiley & Sons Ltd. Published 2021 by John Wiley & Sons Ltd.
Companion website: www.wiley.com/go/foxhall/oral-health-education

4   What are the four main oral health messages?
   A Reduce the consumption of sugar and especially the frequency that food and drinks containing sugar are consumed; clean the teeth and gums thoroughly every day with fluoride toothpaste; fluoride; and dental radiographs
   B Reduce the consumption of sugar and especially the frequency that food and drinks containing sugar are consumed; clean the teeth and gums thoroughly every day with fluoride toothpaste; regular dental attendance; and fluoride
   C Reduce the consumption of sugar and especially the frequency that food and drinks containing sugar are consumed; clean the teeth and gums thoroughly every day with fluoride toothpaste; regular dental attendance; and emergency dental intervention and specialist care
   D Reduce the consumption of sugar and especially the frequency that food and drinks containing sugar are consumed; clean the teeth at least once a day and use mouthwash; regular dental attendance; and fluoride

5   Studies from Tannahill cover three main areas, what are these?
   A Prevention, health assessment, and health education
   B Prevention, health promotion, and health education
   C Prevention, health promotion, and healthcare
   D Prevention, health promotion, and sharing ideas with others
   E Seek advice from a dentist, health promotion, and health education

6   What does BSPD stand for?
   A British Society of Paediatric Dental Assistance
   B British Society of Paediatric Dentists
   C British Society of Paediatric Dentistry
   D Britain's Society of Periodontal Dentistry
   E Basic State of Periodontal Dentistry

7   In a study on how the public learns, Tones K suggests the success of health education is dependent on persuasion. What does this theory ignore?
   A Diet advice
   B Healthier options
   C Oral health education
   D Persuasion skills
   E Social background of ill health

8   Many studies have been carried out on how the public learn theories of health. What theory were Prochaska and DiClemente responsible for?
   A Study of persuasion to change to healthier options
   B Study of procrastination with young adults
   C Study of prevention, health protection, and health education
   D Study of the process of change
   E Study of voluntary actions to promote oral health education

Extended Matching Questions

For each of the following questions, select the most appropriate answer from the list below. The answers might be used once, more than once, or not at all.

Topic: Oral Health Messages

a) Brushing 2 × daily with fluoride toothpaste
b) Diet sheet
c) Fruit and vegetable snacks
d) Fluoride treatment
e) High caries risk
f) Interdental brushes
g) Questionnaire
h) Regular dental attendance

1   You have a 12-year-old male patient booked in for his second oral health education session regarding his fixed orthodontic appliance. The dentist would like you to focus on the oral health message 'clean the teeth and gums thoroughly every day with fluoride toothpaste'. You reinforce your advice from the first session which included toothbrushing twice a day with a fluoride toothpaste. From the list above select one other oral hygiene aid you can suggest to help improve his plaque control?

2   You have a 32-year-old female booked in for an oral health education session regarding her high caries risk. She has not seen a dentist regularly for the past 18 years. She admits she has an extremely poor diet of high sugary snacks and fruit juice. Which of the answers from the list would be the most appropriate step in your first appointment together to create a plan for the patient's sessions?

3   You have an 8-year-old female patient booked in for an oral health education session regarding brushing techniques. The mother and father show little knowledge of dental hygiene. You are making your lesson plan the night before. Which of the answers from the list would be the most appropriate piece of information to provide this patient during the first session?

Answers

1 A nursing mother has attended the dental practice for oral hygiene advice; which of the following pieces of advice would you not recommend?

Correct Answer: c) For the baby to use a dummy, dip the dummy in jam

This would not be recommended for any child or baby. Jam is a high-sugar food which can contribute to caries.

2 The four key oral health messages were put in place for dental health education. When seeing a patient for an educational session you should provide information from one message per session. Today, you are focusing on the message 'reduce the consumptions of sugar the frequency of intake of food and drink containing sugar'. Which of the following pieces of information is not included in either of the four oral health messages?

Correct Answer: d) The prescription and timings of the dental radiographs

The four oral health messages cover diet, toothbrushing instructions, dental attendance, and fluoride. They do not cover prescriptions and timings of dental radiographs, recall intervals leading to ongoing treatments, and emergency dental interventions between episodes of specialist care.

3 Oral health messages are provided by many people; it should be imperative that the messages given are all the same to stop confusion. Who out of the following would not provide and support oral health messages?

Correct Answer: e) Police

The police would not provide and/or support oral health messages; usually these would be covered by healthcare professionals only.

4 What are the four main oral health messages?

Correct Answer: b) Reduce the consumption of sugar and especially the frequency that food and drinks containing sugar are consumed; clean the teeth and gums thoroughly every day with fluoride toothpaste; regular dental attendance; and fluoride

The four main oral health messages should always be conveyed to patients; only one of the messages should be covered per session and then they can be evaluated at the following session.

5 Studies from Tannahill cover three main areas, what are these?

Correct Answer: b) Prevention, health promotion, and health education

A Tannahill model of health promotion concerns three main areas: prevention, health promotion, and health education. Tannahill covered all healthcare and promoted general well-being.

6   What does BSPD stand for?

Correct Answer: c) British Society of Paediatric Dentistry

The British Society for Paediatric Dentistry is the national society is specifically concerned with the oral health of children in the UK.

7   The study on how the public learns, Tones K suggests the success of health education is dependent on persuasion. What does this theory ignore?

Correct Answer: e) Social background of ill health

In the study, Tones K suggests that the health educator would be successful based on persuasion to choose a healthier option. This theory ignores the socio-economic or social background of ill health.

8   Many studies have been carried out on how the public learn theories of health. What theory were Prochaska and DiClemente responsible for?

Correct Answer: d) Study of the process of change

Prochaska and DiClemente's study describes the process of change. It suggests that individuals may be at one of a number of stages in relation to making a lifestyle change:

1) Pre-contemplation – patients are not thinking about changing their behaviour; they are not aware that they have a problem and are likely to resist any pressure to change.
2) Contemplation – patients are aware that they have a problem and realise that they must do something about it, but have not yet made a commitment to change in the near future.
3) Preparation – patients begin to make small behavioural changes and make a commitment to take action in the near future.
4) Action – patients take action to alter their behaviour.
5) Maintenance – patients continue their efforts towards achieving a permanent change.

This study also suggests that patients' motivation may vary. When change is self-initiated it is more likely to be successful. Whole processes or parts of them may be repeated several times before permanent change is achieved.

Extended Matching Questions

Topic: Oral Health Messages

1   You have a 12-year-old male patient booked in for his second oral health education session regarding his fixed orthodontic appliance. The dentist would like you to focus on the oral health message 'clean the teeth and gums thoroughly every day with fluoride toothpaste', You reinforce your advice from the first session which included toothbrushing twice a day with a fluoride toothpaste. From the list above select one other oral hygiene aid you can suggest to help improve his plaque control?

Correct Answer: d) Interdental brushes

A patient who has a fixed orthodontic appliance must understand that not only is cleaning his teeth with fluoride toothpaste important, but to also clean under the arch wires to prevent plaque and food debris collecting. If food debris and plaque are not removed daily, then it can lead to staining and cavities when the appliance is removed.

2   You have a 32-year-old female booked in for an oral health education session regarding her high caries risk. She has not seen a dentist regularly for the past 18 years. She admits she has an extremely poor diet of high sugary snacks and fruit juice. Which of the answers from the list would be the most appropriate step in your first appointment together to create a plan for the patient's sessions?

Correct Answer: b) Diet sheet

When you are meeting with a patient for the first time, in order to work out which oral health messages you need to provide the patient you will need to get an idea of her current diet and her current knowledge. If you are aware that she already has a poor diet, then completing a diet sheet with her will give you a good understanding of when she is consuming sugary foods or drinks and then you can apply your knowledge on how to adapt the diet to be healthier.

3   You have an 8-year-old female patient booked in for an oral health education session regarding brushing techniques. The mother and father show little knowledge of dental hygiene. You are making your lesson plan the night before. Which of the answers from the list would be the most appropriate piece of information to provide this patient during the first session?

Correct Answer: a) Brushing 2 × daily with fluoride toothpaste

It is common that children do not like to brush their teeth, and if they are, then they aren't doing it correctly. In the first session it may be a good idea to cover how the patient is brushing and, if the technique is incorrect, then show the patient and the parents the correct techniques. You may also need to provide advice on toothpaste with adequate fluoride.

2

Eruption

1   What is the average eruption date for a permanent lower central incisor?
   A 5–7 years
   B 6–7 years
   C 6–8 years
   D 8–10 years
   E 12–13 years

2   What is the average eruption date for a permanent upper first molar?
   A 6–7 years
   B 6–8 years
   C 7–9 years
   D 10–11 years
   E 12–13 years

3   What is the average eruption date for a permanent upper second premolar?
   A 7–8 years
   B 9–11 years
   C 10–11 years
   D 10–12 years
   E 12–13 years

4   What is the average eruption date for a permanent lower third molar?
   A 16–22 years
   B 17–25 years
   C 18–19 years
   D 18–21 years
   E 18–25 years

Questions and Answers in Oral Health Education, First Edition. Chloe Foxhall and Anna Lown.
© 2021 John Wiley & Sons Ltd. Published 2021 by John Wiley & Sons Ltd.
Companion website: www.wiley.com/go/foxhall/oral-health-education

5 What is the average eruption date in months for a deciduous lower first molar?
   A 12 months
   B 14 months
   C 16 months
   D 18 months
   E 20 months

6 What is the average eruption date in months for a deciduous lower canine?
   A 6 months
   B 14 months
   C 15 months
   D 20 months
   E 24 months

7 What is the average eruption date in months for a deciduous upper central incisor?
   A 8 months
   B 10 months
   C 12 months
   D 20 months
   E 22 months

8 What is the average eruption date in months for a deciduous upper second molar?
   A 12 months
   B 24 months
   C 27 months
   D 29 months
   E 30 months

9 You are asked to give oral health advice on toothbrushing to a parent and child. The child is 3 years' old. What dentition would you presume to be present at this age?
   A All central incisors, lateral incisors, and canines
   B All deciduous dentition
   C Central incisors, lateral incisors, and second molars
   D Central incisors, lateral incisors, canines, and first molars
   E Lateral incisors, canines and first molars

10 You are asked to give oral health advice on diet to a parent of a 1 year old. What dentition would you presume to be present at this age?
   A Central incisors and first molars
   B Central incisors and second molars
   C Lower central incisors and canines
   D Upper and lower central incisors and upper lateral incisors
   E Upper and lower central incisors, canines and first molars

Extended Matching Questions

For each of the following questions select the most appropriate answer from the list below. The answers might be used once, more than once, or not at all.

Topic: Eruption

a) Cutting and biting into food
b) Ripping and tearing food
c) 4 canines and 4 molars
d) 6 to 7
e) 8 incisors
f) 12 teeth
g) 10 to 12
h) 18 to 25

1 A 13-year-old female has attended the dental practice today for a dental examination; she is missing her lower left canine. The dentist has taken a radiography and confirms that as the patient is missing the lower left canine. The patient may suffer some loss of function. Which of the answers would be the most appropriate for the function she may lose?

2 A patient has attended an oral health session with you today, and at the end of the session the patient asks for some advice about her 1-year-old child. The patient is concerned about how many teeth they have as they are struggling to eat soft foods like bread and banana. Which of the answers is most appropriate to explain how many teeth the child most likely would have at that age?

Answers

1 What is the average eruption date for a permanent lower central incisor?

Correct Answer: b) 6–7 years

The average eruption date for a permanent lower central incisor to erupt is around 6–7 years of age.

2 What is the average eruption date for a permanent upper first molar?

Correct Answer: a) 6–7 years

The average eruption date for a permanent upper first molar erupts around 6–7 years of age.

3 What is the average eruption date for a permanent upper second premolar?

Correct Answer: c) 10–11 years

The average eruption date for a permanent upper second molar to erupt is around 10–11 years.

4 What is the average eruption date for a permanent lower third molar?

Correct Answer: e) 18–25 years

The average eruption date for a permanent lower third molar to erupt is around 18–25 years.

5 What is the average eruption date in months for a deciduous lower first molar?

Correct Answer: c) 16 months

The average eruption date in months for a deciduous lower first molar to erupt is around 16 months.

6 What is the average eruption date in months for a deciduous lower canine?

Correct Answer: d) 20 months

The average eruption date in months for a deciduous lower canine is around 20 months.

7 What is the average eruption date in months for a deciduous upper central incisor?

Correct Answer: b) 10 months

The average eruption date in months for a deciduous upper central incisor is around 10 months.

8 What is the average eruption date in months for a deciduous upper second molar?

Correct Answer: d) 29 months

The average eruption date in months for a deciduous upper second molar is around 29 months.

9 You are asked to give oral health advice on toothbrushing to a parent and child. The child is 3 years' old. What dentition would you presume to be present at this age?

Correct Answer: b) All deciduous dentition

At age 3 (36 months), all deciduous dentition should be present.

10 You are asked to give oral health advice on diet to a parent of a 1 year old. What dentition would you presume to be present at this age?

Correct Answer: d) Upper and lower central incisors and upper lateral incisors

At age 1 (12 months) the upper and lower central incisors and upper lateral incisors should be present.

Extended Matching Questions

Topic: Eruption

1 A 13-year-old female has attended the dental practice today for a dental examination; she is missing her lower left canine. The dentist has taken a radiography and confirms that as the patient is missing the lower left canine. The patient may suffer some loss of function. Which of the answers would be the most appropriate for the function she may lose?

Correct Answer: b) Ripping and tearing food

The canines provide the ripping and tearing function when eating; this function is especially good when eating tough foods like meat. The upper canines erupt around the age of 9 or 10 and the lower canines erupt around the age of 10–12. These ages can vary slightly depending on the patient.

2 A patient has attended an oral health session with you today; at the end of the session the patient asks for some advice about her 1-year-old child. The patient is concerned about how many teeth they have as they are struggling to eat soft foods like bread and banana. Which of the answers is most appropriate to explain how many teeth the child most likely would have at that age?

Correct Answer: f) 12 teeth

A 1-year-old would most likely be in the middle stages of having the deciduous teeth erupt. The 4 central incisors would erupt around 6 months. The 4 lateral incisors would erupt around 8 months. The 4 first molars would erupt around 12 months, the 4 canines would erupt around 18 months, and then the second molars would erupt around 24 months.

3

Anatomy and the Oral Mucosa

1   In a tooth, what surrounds the outside of the pulp chamber?
    A Cementum
    B Dentine
    C Enamel
    D Gingiva
    E Periodontal ligament

2   How long after the tooth eruption does the root fully form?
    A 1 years
    B 2 years
    C 3 years
    D 4 years
    E 5 years

3   What are the two most common inorganic constituents in enamel?
    A Calcium and phosphate
    B Collagen fibres and phosphate
    C Hydroxyapatite and fluor apatite
    D Salt and water
    E Salt and fluor apatite

4   Enamel structure consists of five things. The first four are: Prisms, incremental lines, lamellae, and tufts. What is the fifth?
    A Amelodentinal junction
    B Bacteria
    C Calcium
    D Crestal
    E Proteins

Questions and Answers in Oral Health Education, First Edition. Chloe Foxhall and Anna Lown.
© 2021 John Wiley & Sons Ltd. Published 2021 by John Wiley & Sons Ltd.
Companion website: www.wiley.com/go/foxhall/oral-health-education

5 What is cementum?

A A bone-like structure that is softer than dentine; it is an attachment for the fibres

B An attachment to the tooth that holds it in place; it also acts as a shock absorber for the tooth

C Cementum makes up the bulk of the tooth; it is softer than enamel and consists of tubules

D Cementum contains nerves and blood vessels; this is the sensory part of the tooth

E It is the fluid which bathes the surfaces of our teeth

6 An elderly patient presents with multiple root caries; the medical history shows the patient has Sjogren's syndrome. What is the most likely reason this would cause cavities?

A Bacteria

B Diet

C Hypersalivation

D Vomiting

E Xerostomia

7 The cranium is made up of several bony plates that form the skull which protects the brain and provides support to many muscles. Which bone supports the masseter muscle?

A Coronoid process

B Maxilla

C Nasal bone

D Zygomatic arch

E Zygomatic bone

8 There are 12 pairs of cranial nerves, which supply movement and sensations in the head and neck. Which pair of nerves supply the teeth and surrounding soft tissues and the muscles of mastication?

A Facial nerve

B Glossopharyngeal nerve

C Hypoglossal nerve

D Long buccal nerve

E Trigeminal nerve

9 A patient attends the dental surgery for a pain in her jaw. On examination, the clinician finds wear on the incisal surfaces of the central incisors and canines. Which type of tooth wear would this be?

A Abfraction

B Abrasion

C Attrition

D Cavitation

E Erosion

10 A Dentist wants to extract the upper right second premolar. Which of the following nerves would be anaesthetised?
A Anterior superior dental nerve
B Lingual nerve
C Long buccal nerve
D Middle superior dental nerve
E Posterior superior dental nerve

11 A Dentist wants to place a restoration of the lower left second molar mesial occlusal. Which of the following nerves would be anaesthetised?
A Inferior dental nerve
B Inferior dental nerve
C Long buccal nerve
D Naso-palatine nerve
E Posterior superior dental nerve

12 There are four major muscles of mastication that are responsible for the forwards, sidewards, and closing movements of the lower jaw. All of these functions are what make us able to chew and speak. Which of the following nerves provides their innervation from the motor branch?
A Facial
B Inferior dental nerve
C Long buccal nerve
D Mandibular
E Mandible

Extended Matching Questions

For each of the following questions select the most appropriate answer from the list below. The answers might be used once, more than once, or not at all.

Topic: Anatomy and the Oral Mucosa

a) Alveolar process
b) Collagen fibres
c) Dentine
d) Enamel
e) Inferior dental nerve
f) Long buccal nerve
g) Odontoblasts
h) Ramus

1 Teeth begin to develop and are present in the jawbone before a baby is born. They are made up of different tissue layers, which are produced or formed by different cells throughout development. Which of the answers is a tooth tissue that continues to develop throughout a patient's life?

2 Teeth are held in the socket by supporting structures that make up the periodontium – most commonly known to include the periodontal ligament, alveolar bone, and gingiva. Which of the answers is the tissue that forms the periodontal ligament?

3 Teeth are held in the socket by supporting structures that make up the periodontium – most commonly known to include the periodontal ligament and gingiva. Which of the answers is the bone that forms the socket?

4 A 26-year-old patient attends the dental practice for crown preparation for the lower right first molar. To ensure the patient has the procedure completed painlessly, which of the options is the nerve that should be anaesthetised for the procedure?

Answers

1 In a tooth, what surrounds the outside of the pulp chamber?

Correct Answer: b) Dentine

Dentine is the main bulk of the tooth and occupies the interior of the crown and root. It surrounds the pulp chamber. It is covered by enamel in the crown of the tooth. It consists of up to 80% inorganic tissue, mainly calcium hydroxyapatite crystals, which are formed by hollow tubes.

2 How long after the tooth eruption does the root fully form?

Correct Answer: c) 3 years

When a tooth is formed in the maxilla or mandible, the root is not fully formed. Only up to around 3 years after the tooth erupts does the root fully form. The apical foramen doesn't close until after the root is fully formed.

3 What are the two most common inorganic constituents in enamel?

Correct Answer: a) Calcium and phosphate

Enamel is the protective outer covering of the crown of a tooth which is highly calcified. It can vary in shade of colour and is the hardest substance in the body. Enamel is made up of 96% mineral crystals, which are inorganic and are arranged in prisms in an organic matrix called the interprismatic substance. The main mineral crystals are calcium hydroxyapatite. The enamel joins the dentine in layers; the junction that connects these two is called the amelodentinal junction.

4 Enamel structure consists of five things. The first four are: Prisms, incremental lines, lamellae, and tufts. What is the fifth?

Correct Answer: a) Amelodentinal junction

The amelodentinal junction is the joint between the enamel and dentine. If caries spread from the enamel to the dentine. They can spread rapidly through the dentine and come close to the pulp chamber.

5 What is cementum?

Correct Answer: a) A bone-like structure that is softer than dentine; it is an attachment for the fibres.

Cementum is the calcified protective outer covering of the root and has a similar structure to bone. Cementum meets the enamel of the tooth at the neck and normally lies beneath the gingivae. Around 65% is mineralised with calcium hydroxyapatite crystals. These lie within a matrix of fibrous tissues with the ends of collagen fibres from the periodontal ligament inserted into the outer layer of the cementum.

6 An elderly patient presents with multiple root caries; the medical history shows the patient has Sjogren's syndrome. What is the most likely reason this would cause cavities?

Correct Answer: e) Xerostomia

Xerostomia is an uncomfortable condition which leads to a constantly dry mouth caused by a decreased production of saliva. Sjogren's syndrome is a syndrome that occurs in conjunction with an autoimmune disorder, such as rheumatoid arthritis. The body's defence system begins to attack itself and destroys its own glandular tissues, which includes salivary glands.

7 The cranium is made up of several bony plates that form the skull which protects the brain and provides support to many muscles. Which bone supports the masseter muscle?

Correct Answer: d) Zygomatic arch

The zygomatic arch is supported by the zygomatic bone and is situated under the eye socket (orbital). The pair of facial bones articulate with the cranium posteriorly and extend anteriorly into the zygomatic arch to articulate the maxilla.

8 There are 12 pairs of cranial nerves, which supply movement and sensations in the head and neck. Which pair of nerves supply the teeth and surrounding soft tissues and the muscles of mastication?

Correct Answer: e) Trigeminal nerve

The trigeminal nerve distributes all of the nerve that supplies the teeth and muscles of the oral cavity. The trigeminal nerve runs down the side of the face and divides into three divisions: ophthalmic, maxillary, and mandibular. These then divide into nerves that would be anaesthetised for dental treatment.

9 A patient attends the dental surgery for a pain in her jaw. On examination, the clinician finds wear on the incisal surfaces of the central incisors and canines. Which type of tooth wear would this be?

Correct Answer: c) Attrition

Attrition is tooth wear, usually on the occlusal and incisal surfaces, that is non-carious. It is caused by bruxism (clenching and grinding) of the teeth. The wear is usually most noticeable on the canines and incisors; they can look worn down to the same height and usually have flat surfaces that meet together with the opposing teeth.

10 A Dentist wants to extract the upper right second premolar, which of the following nerves would be anaesthetised?

Correct Answer: d) Middle superior dental nerve

The middle superior dental nerve supplies the buccal side of the maxillary premolars and the mesial half of the upper first molar. The greater palatine nerve would also be anaesthetised. This supplies the palate of the maxillary molars and premolars.

11 A dentist wants to place a restoration of the lower left second molar mesial occlusal; which of the following nerves would be anaesthetised?

Correct Answer: b) Inferior dental nerve

The technique to anaesthitise the inferior dental nerve is known as an ID block, it is given to anaesthetise the mandibular premolars and molars' pulp and investing structures.

12 There are four muscles of mastication which are responsible for the forwards, sidewards, and closing movements of the lower jaw. All of these functions are what make us able to chew and speak. Which of the following nerves provides their innervation from the motor branch?

Correct Answer: d) Mandibular

The trigeminal nerve separates into three divisions, one of which is the mandibular division. The other two are the maxilla and the ophthalmic division. The mandibular division has a motor branch which innervates the muscles of mastication. The motor branch supplies stimulation to the muscles of mastication to create chewing movements.

Extended Matching Questions

Topic: Anatomy and the Oral Mucosa

1 Teeth begin to develop and are present in the jawbone before a baby is born. They are made up of different tissue layers, which are produced or formed by different cells throughout development. Which of the answers is a tooth tissue that continues to develop throughout a patient's life?

Correct Answer: c) Dentine

Dentine is the tooth tissue that can continue to develop throughout a patient's life. Dentine is formed by odontoblasts which lie along the amelodentinal junction of the tooth's structure. Dentine can develop into secondary dentine when responding to pain or caries in order to protect the pulp from trauma or infection. Dentine can also develop with age, which is why it is generally harder to complete a root canal treatment on an elderly patient, because the pulp chamber becomes smaller with time.

2 Teeth are held in the socket by supporting structures that make up the periodontium – most commonly known to include the periodontal ligament, alveolar bone, and gingiva. Which of the answers is the tissue that forms the periodontal ligament?

Correct Answer: b) Collagen fibres

Collagen is protein originally formed from fibroblasts and forms a type of connective tissue. The fibres attach the cementum to the alveolar bone or dental soft tissues to allow a cushion for the tooth to push onto during chewing or biting. The periodontal ligament is seen as a shock absorber for the tooth; if trauma is caused to a tooth the biting or chewing action, it can cause pain which comes from the periodontal ligament.

3 Teeth are held in the socket by supporting structures that make up the periodontium – most commonly known to include the periodontal ligament and gingiva. Which of the answers is the bone that forms the socket?

Correct Answer: a) Alveolar process

The alveolar process is the thickened ridge of bone that supports the teeth. The alveolar process can be lost through resorption caused by disease and extraction.

4 A 26-year-old patient attends the dental practice for crown preparation for the lower right first molar. To ensure the patient has the procedure completed painlessly, which of the options is the nerve that should be anaesthetised for the procedure?

Correct Answer: e) Inferior dental nerve

The inferior dental nerve supplies all the molar teeth on the lower jaw. It is a branch of the mandibular nerve which is a branch on the trigeminal nerve (the fifth cranial nerve). It is the largest nerve on the mandible. It is situated inside the body of the mandible and exits through the mental foramen which is between the roots of the lower premolars.

4

Saliva

1   The mouth contains three main salivary glands which produce saliva at various rates. From the following, what are the three major salivary glands?
    A Parotid, Submandibular, and Sublingual
    B Stenson's, Submandibular, and Sublingual
    C Sublingual, Parotid duct, and Buccinator
    D Sublingual, Submandibular, and Stenson's
    E Wharton's, Stenson's, and Parotid

2   The salivary glands are spread out around the mouth, this means that all areas of the mouth can be well lubricated. Where is the parotid salivary gland situated?
    A Below the mylohyoid line, against the body of the mandible
    B In the posterior region of the floor of the mouth
    C Lies at the floor of the mouth, above the mylohyoid line
    D On the inside of the mandible
    E Over the outside and partly behind the ramus of the mandible, in front of the ear

3   The digestive enzyme present in saliva is also known as?
    A Antibodies
    B Immunoglobulins
    C Leucocytes
    D Mucus
    E Salivary amylase

4   What are the two types of cell found in the salivary glands?
    A Antibacterial enzymes and mucous
    B Antibodies and leukocytes
    C Minerals and sodium
    D Mucous secretory cells and serous secretory cells
    E Ptyalin and mucous

Questions and Answers in Oral Health Education, First Edition. Chloe Foxhall and Anna Lown.
© 2021 John Wiley & Sons Ltd. Published 2021 by John Wiley & Sons Ltd.
Companion website: www.wiley.com/go/foxhall/oral-health-education

5 The mouth's pH level changes throughout the day due to food and drink; what is generally considered neutral pH balance of the mouth?

A pH 4

B pH 5

C pH 6

D pH 7

E pH 9

6 When an acid attack occurs through consumption of acidic food, the pH level will adjust leaving the teeth at risk. What level does the pH need to fall below for enamel demineralisation to occur?

A 5

B 5.5

C 6

D 6.8

E 7

7 A patient has noticed that they have less saliva than they used to. The dentist wants to give the patient a full explanation that less saliva can have serious consequences; from the following options, what are the main serious consequences?

A Caries, poor taste sensation, oral infections, oral soft tissue trauma, and problems with speech and mastication

B Caries, speech, mastication, and poor taste

C Oral cancer and caries

D Periodontal disease and caries

E Periodontal disease, caries, oral cancer, and soft tissue trauma

8 A patient attends the dental practice for some advice, the patient is diagnosed with Ptyalism. What is Ptyalism?

A A hereditary form of xerostomia

B Bad breath

C Bad tasting saliva

D Excessive salivation

E Too little saliva

9 A patient attends the dental practice for her six-monthly appointment for an exam. She completes an updated medical history form. The patient complains of having a dry mouth which makes it hard for her to keep her denture in place. What can cause xerostomia?

A Irradiation, Sjogren's syndrome, and medications

B Medications

C Not brushing teeth as required

D Trauma

E Wearing a denture

Extended Matching Questions

For each of the following questions, select the most appropriate answer from the list below. The answers might be used once, more than once or not at all.

Topic: Saliva

a) Cleaning the teeth along with the lips, tongue, and cheeks.
b) Hyper salivation
c) Inorganic salts and organic collagen fibres
d) Liver disease
e) Protein and waste products
f) Serotonin syndrome
g) Sjogren's syndrome
h) Xerostomia

1 Saliva is the oral fluid which bathes the surfaces of our teeth. Saliva is made up of 99.5% water and 0.5% dissolved substances. Which of the answers is the most appropriate one for what is included in the dissolved substances?

2 Saliva is the oral fluid which bathes the surfaces of our teeth. Saliva has multiple uses in the oral cavity. Which of the answers is the most appropriate for one of the functions of saliva?

3 A 68-year-old patient attends the dental practice for an emergency appointment. They have asked to discuss a problem they are experiencing following a medical diagnosis they received from the doctor. The patient has experienced a dry mouth and halitosis. She has also suffered from fatigue and muscle soreness. Which of the answers is most appropriate to which medical diagnosis she has received based on the effects she has experienced?

Answers

1   The mouth contains three main salivary glands which produce saliva at various rates. From the following, select the three major salivary glands?

    Correct Answer: a) Parotid, Submandibular, and Sublingual

    The Parotid, Submandibular, and Sublingual glands are all present in the oral cavity. The Parotid gland is situated between the ramus and mandible of the ear. The Submandibular gland is situated in the posterior area of the floor of the mouth, beneath the mylohyoid muscle. The Sublingual gland is situated in the anterior area of the floor of the mouth, just above the mylohyoid muscle.

2   The salivary glands are spread out around the mouth; this means that all areas of the mouth can be well lubricated. Where is the parotid salivary gland situated?

    Correct Answer: e) Over the outside and partly behind the ramus of the mandible, in front of the ear

    The parotid gland is situated between the ramus and mandible of the ear.

3   The digestive enzyme present in saliva is also known as?

    Correct Answer: e) Salivary amylase

    Salivary amylase is a digestive enzyme otherwise known as ptyalin. It initiates starch digestion, before the food is swallowed.

4   What are the two types of cell found in the salivary glands?

    Correct Answer: d) Mucous secretory cells and serous secretory cells

    Mucous secretory cells produce a thick substance which aids lubrication in the mouth. It contains enzymes and minerals.
    Serous secretory cells produce a thin substance containing antibodies and electrolytes.

5   The mouth's pH level changes throughout the day due to food and drink; what is generally considered neutral pH balance of the mouth?

    Correct Answer: d) pH 7

    The pH balance of the mouth is slightly alkaline, at pH 7; this is due to the electrolyte components present in it.

6   When an acid attack occurs through consumption of acidic food, the pH level will adjust leaving the teeth at risk. What level does the pH need to fall below for enamel demineralisation to occur?

    Correct Answer: b) 5.5

    If the pH balance falls below 5.5 then this is classed as a critical level. At this stage, enamel demineralisation will occur and potentially lead to a cavity.

7 A patient has noticed that they have less saliva than they used to. The dentist wants to give the patient a full explanation that less saliva can have serious consequences. From the following options, what are the main serious consequences?

Correct Answer: a) Caries, poor taste sensation, oral infections, oral soft tissue trauma, and problems with speech and mastication

A reduction in saliva can cause many serious problems. The patient will be more susceptible to dental caries as the self-cleaning ability is lost. They will not enjoy their food as much as the taste buds cannot function correctly. They will be more at risk of oral infections as the capability to defend the oral environment is reduced. The risk of soft tissue trauma is also increased as saliva is a protective mechanism and this is reduced. Finally, the patient's speech and ability to eat will be affected. The patient will find it difficult to speak and eat normally as the saliva is a much needed lubricant, and this will be reduced.

8 A patient attends the dental practice for some advice, the patient is diagnosed with Ptyalism. What is Ptyalism?

Correct Answer: d) Excessive salivation

Ptyalism is excessive salivation where a patient will produce more saliva than needed. The condition could be linked to a disease.

9 A patient attends the dental practice for her six-monthly appointment for an exam. She completes an updated medical history form. The patient complains of having a dry mouth which makes it hard for her to keep her denture in place. What can cause Xerostomia?

Correct Answer: a) Irradiation, Sjogren's syndrome, and medications

Irradiation of the head and neck area, usually because of radiotherapy for cancer in this area. Sjogren's syndrome that occurs in conjunction with an autoimmune disorder. This is where the body's defence system attacks itself and destroys its own glandular tissues.

Extended Matching Questions

Topic: Saliva

1 Saliva is the oral fluid which bathes the surfaces of our teeth. Saliva is made up of 99.5% water and 0.5% dissolved substances. Which of the answers is the most appropriate one for what is included in the dissolved substances?

Correct Answer: e) Protein and waste products

Saliva is made up of 99.5% water and 0.5% dissolved substances. The dissolved substances include protein and waste products. The protein contains mucoid, enzymes, and serum proteins. The waste products contain inorganic ions and gases. When saliva enters the mouth, viruses, bacteria, yeast, remains of food and drink, and leukocytes are added.

2 Saliva is the oral fluid which bathes the surfaces of our teeth. Saliva has multiple uses in the oral cavity. Which of the answers is the most appropriate for one of the functions of saliva?

Correct Answer: a) Cleaning the teeth along with the lips, tongue, and cheeks

The functions of saliva are:

- Cleaning the teeth along with the lips, tongue, and cheeks.
- Lubricates the food bolus to help it slip down the throat.
- It breaks down the cooked starch through the enzyme salivary amylase which is contained in the saliva.
- Accelerates blood coagulation.
- Neutralises acid creating a buffer action with the presence of bicarbonate ions in the saliva.
- Helps with speech.
- Helps dissolve food to allow taste buds to work.
- Water balance.

3 A 68-year-old patient attends the dental practice for an emergency appointment. They have asked to discuss a problem they are experiencing following a medical diagnosis they received from the doctor. The patient has experienced a dry mouth and halitosis. She has also suffered from fatigue and muscle soreness. Which of the answers is most appropriate to which medical diagnosis she has received based on the effects she has experienced?

Correct Answer: g) Sjogren's syndrome

Sjogren's syndrome is a condition that affects the parts of the body that produce fluid such as the eyes and the mouth. Some of the symptoms can be:

- dry eyes
- dry mouth
- halitosis
- fatigue
- muscle soreness.

There is currently no cure for Sjogren's syndrome. Advice should be given on how to continue living a relatively normal lifestyle. Products like artificial saliva are available for patients that suffer with xerostomia.

5

Periodontal Disease and Plaque

1 A patient visits the practice for an assessment. After a full examination, including a basic periodontal examination and some periapicals being taken, the patient is diagnosed with periodontal disease. What causes periodontal disease?
   A Plaque
   B Plaque, medical conditions, and time
   C Plaque, refined carbohydrates, and time
   D Poor oral hygiene and plaque build-up along the gingival margin
   E Sugars

2 When diagnosing a patient with periodontal disease, the dentist has to look at all contributing factors. From the answers below select the most comprehensive list of contributing factors for periodontal disease?
   A HPV, diabetes, and weakened immune system
   B Pregnancy and smoking
   C Smoking, diabetes, pregnancy, and a weakened immune system
   D Smoking, pregnancy, and a poor diet
   E Smoking, medication, and HPV

3 Can a patient taking a medication that causes xerostomia be more at risk of developing periodontal disease?
   A It depends on the medication name
   B It depends on the strength of the medication
   C It only makes a difference if the medication is taken daily
   D No, it will not make a difference which medication the patient is taking
   E Yes, medication can be a contributing factor

4 A patient attends the dental practice for an exam appointment. During the basic periodontal examination, the patient presents with a BPE of 3 in two sextants of the mouth; what does this mean?
   A The teeth in those quadrants have furcation
   B The teeth in those quadrants have gross caries
   C The teeth in those quadrants have a probing depth of between 3.5 and 5.5 mm
   D The teeth in those quadrants have a probing depth of between 0 and 3 mm
   E The teeth in those quadrants are mobile and have a pocket depth of 3 mm

Questions and Answers in Oral Health Education, First Edition. Chloe Foxhall and Anna Lown.
© 2021 John Wiley & Sons Ltd. Published 2021 by John Wiley & Sons Ltd.
Companion website: www.wiley.com/go/foxhall/oral-health-education

5   A patient attends the dental practice for an exam appointment. During the basic periodontal examination, the patient presents with a BPE code *; what does this suggest?
   A   The patient has bone loss and requires oral health instructions and root surface debridement
   B   The patient has extensive bone loss and pockets of above 5.5 mm in depth that require a chlorhexidine mouthwash
   C   The patient has furcation involvement and requires diet advice
   D   The patient has furcation involvement and requires oral health instructions and root surface debridement and possible referral
   E   The patient has gross caries

6   What do the letters BPE stand for?
   A   Basic periodontal examination
   B   Basic periodontal ligament examination
   C   Brilliant periodontal exam
   D   Black banded periodontal exam
   E   Bleeding periodontal examination

7   A patient has attended the surgery for an exam appointment. The dentist sends a referral to the oral health educator and the oral hygienist. In the clinical notes from the exam appointment, the dentist states the patient had three signs of gingivitis. From the options below, which would be the most suitable answer?
   A   Loss of stippling, swelling, redness
   B   Loss of stippling, pain, heat
   C   Swelling, sensitivity, pain
   D   Redness, heat, bleeding
   E   Redness, bleeding, pain

8   When there is a collection of plaque around a tooth or area of the mouth, what is this called?
   A   Dental caries
   B   Fissure stagnation area
   C   Gingival margin biofilm
   D   Plaque biofilm area
   E   Stagnation area

9   Calculus is the hard rock-like deposit commonly seen on the lingual surface of the lower incisors. What are the two factors necessary for its formation?
   A   Plaque and food debris
   B   Plaque and toxins
   C   Saliva and food debris
   D   Saliva and plaque
   E   Stagnation areas and plaque

10 A patient presents with chronic gingivitis and requires oral health advice. What advice would you give the patient?

    A Reduce sugar consumption

    B Reduce sugar consumption and use a fluoride mouthwash

    C Remove all plaque by using a fluoridated toothpaste and soft/medium textured toothbrush, alongside interdental cleaning

    D Take prescribed antibiotics

    E Use a chlorhexidine mouthwash

Extended Matching Questions

For each of the following questions, select the most appropriate answer from the list below. The answers might be used once, more than once or not at all.

Topic: Periodontal disease and Plaque

a) Draining sinus
b) False pocket
c) Halitosis
d) Periodontal abscess
e) True pocket
f) Streptococcus mutans
g) Spirochaete and fusiform
h) Six point pocket chart

1 If plaque is left on the teeth for three days after it has formed, anaerobic bacteria will be present in increasing numbers. Which of the answers is the most appropriate for the name of the bacteria these anaerobic bacteria?

2 A 38-year-old female attends the dental practice for an appointment. The patient complains of sore, painful gums that bleed when they are touched with a toothbrush. The dentist recorded a BPE, the lower anteriors had a code of 3, all other areas had a code of 1s or 2s. The patient admits she cannot use interdental brushes in this area because her teeth are crowded. Which of the answers is the most appropriate for the pocketing the patient has on the lower anteriors?

3 Periodontal disease gradually destroys the periodontal membrane and the bone supporting the teeth. A pocket forms and allows greater build up of food debris and plaque. Which of the answers is the most appropriate for what can form if this is not cleaned regularly?

Answers

1   A patient visits the practice for an assessment; after a full examination including a basic periodontal examination and some periapicals taken, the patient is diagnosed with periodontal disease. What causes periodontal disease?

    Correct Answer: d) Poor oral hygiene and plaque build up along the gingival margin

    Periodontal disease is predominantly caused by poor oral hygiene and accumulation of plaque at the gingival margin. With the accumulation of plaque along the gingival margin leading to enlarged gingival tissues, this results in false gingival pockets. Plaque bacteria accumulate in these pockets and start to destroy the periodontal ligaments and supporting structures, thus leading to tooth mobility and ultimately tooth loss.

2   When diagnosing a patient with periodontal disease, the dentist has to look at all contributing factors. From the answers below select the most comprehensive list of contributing factors for periodontal disease?

    Correct Answer: c) Smoking, diabetes, pregnancy, and a weakened immune system

    Smoking restricts the blood vessels in the oral cavity and thus masks some of the signs of gingivitis. Bleeding gingiva is usually one of the first signs of gingivitis and helps with the detection of the condition.

    Diabetes has a direct link with periodontal disease. One of the most common causes is having high blood sugar levels for a long period of time. Too much sugar in your blood can lead to more sugar in the saliva, which is a breeding ground for bacteria. These bacteria produces acid, which attacks the tooth enamel and damages the gingiva.

3   Can a patient taking a medication that causes xerostomia be more at risk of developing periodontal disease?

    Correct Answer: e) Yes, medication can be a contributing factor

    If a patient takes any medication that causes xerostomia, then there is less saliva in the oral cavity. With limited saliva in the oral cavity, there is less of a buffer action when food is consumed. With the food particles remaining and bacteria present, this will then lead to plaque accumulation and ultimately lead to periodontal disease.

4   A patient attends the dental practice for an exam appointment. During the basic periodontal examination, the patient presents with a BPE of 3 in two sextants of the mouth; what does this mean?

    Correct Answer: c) The teeth in those quadrants have a probing depth of between 3.5 and 5.5 mm

    With a BPE of 3, the probing depth is 3.5–5.5 mm (the black band is partially visible, indicating a pocket of 3.5–5.5 mm). This means that the tooth has bone loss and the patient is suffering from periodontal disease.

5 A patient attends the dental practice for an exam appointment. During the basic periodontal examination, the patient presents with a BPE code *; what does this suggest?

Correct Answer: d) The patient has furcation involvement and requires oral health instructions and root surface debridement and possible referral

If a * has been used when having a BPE performed on a patient, then this indicates that there is furcation involvement. Furcation is when the junction of the roots beneath the crown are exposed.

6 What do the letters BPE stand for?

Correct Answer: a) Basic periodontal examination

BPE stands for basic periodontal examination. This is the screening index for periodontal disease. The BPE does not monitor the disease progression nor can it be used to formulate a treatment plan. It does indicate if a further examination is required, e.g. the six-point pocket chart.

7 A patient has attended the surgery for an exam appointment. The dentist sends a referral to the oral health educator and the oral hygienist. In the clinical notes from the exam appointment, the dentist states the patient had three signs of gingivitis. From the options below, which would be the most suitable answer?

Correct Answer: a) Loss of stippling, swelling, and redness

The gingiva will appear swollen and red in colour, compared to the healthy condition, and the clear stippling appearance will be less obvious.

8 When there is a collection of plaque around a tooth or area of the mouth, what is this called?

Correct Answer: e) Stagnation area

A combination of bacteria and food debris on the tooth surface creates a transparent, protein-containing, sticky, soft film called a plaque biofilm. It tends to form most in areas where it cannot easily be dislodged. These areas could include the fissures, the margins, and around restorations or dentures.

9 Calculus is the hard rock-like deposit commonly seen on the lingual surface of the lower incisors. What are the two factors necessary for its formation?

Correct Answer: d) Saliva and plaque

The two factors necessary for calculus formation are plaque and saliva. When saliva and plaque interact, this produces a deposition of calculus. This can also be known as solidified plaque. Calculus can also be categorised into subgingival calculus (below the gingival margin) and supragingival calculus (above the gingival margin).

10 A patient presents with chronic gingivitis and requires oral health advice. What advice would you give the patient?

Correct Answer: c) Remove all plaque by using a fluoridated toothpaste and soft/medium textured toothbrush, alongside interdental cleaning

If a patient was sent to you for oral health advice, you would need to give advice based on the current condition of the oral health. As the patient presents with chronic gingivitis, they must receive advice about plaque removal to help prevent the condition from progressing to periodontitis. The patient's current oral health status can be reversed with an optimum oral cleaning regime, which would include removing all plaque by using a soft/medium textured toothbrush and also carrying out interdental cleaning. This cleaning regime must be carried out twice daily and regular maintenance and check up visits carried out by the dental care professional to check on progress and stability.

Extended Matching Questions

Topic: Periodontal disease and Plaque

1 If plaque is left on the teeth for three days after it has formed, anaerobic bacteria will be present in increasing numbers. Which of the answers is the most appropriate for the name of the bacteria these anaerobic bacteria?

Correct Answer: g) Spirochete and fusiform

Plaque forms from saliva as a thin film called the salivary pellicle. This forms within a short period of time and will be invaded by streptococcus bacteria. After 24 hours the film starts to form and is visible. After three days, spirochete and fusiform bacteria can be found.

2 A 38-year-old female attends the dental practice for an appointment. The patient complains of sore, painful gums that bleed when they are touched with a toothbrush. The dentist recorded a BPE, the lower anteriors had a code of 3, all other areas had a code of 1s or 2s. The patient admits she cannot use interdental brushes in this area because her teeth are crowded. Which of the answers is the most appropriate for the pocketing the patient has on the lower anteriors?

Correct Answer: b) False pocket

A false pocket is formed after plaque is left on the teeth and gums for 7–14 days. The bacteria penetrate the tissues causing inflammation; the body then increases the blood flow to the inflamed area to try and fight off the bacteria with antibodies and white blood cells. The increased blood flow causes the gingiva to appear red in colour and can appear swollen. The swelling of the gingiva causes the false pocket between the gingiva and the tooth, causing food debris and plaque to become trapped.

3 Periodontal disease gradually destroys the periodontal membrane and the bone supporting the teeth. A pocket forms and allows greater build up of food debris and plaque. Which of the answers is the most appropriate for what can form if this is not cleaned regularly?

Correct Answer: d) Periodontal abscess

Periodontal abscesses are caused by a true pocket containing food debris and plaque. A periodontal abscess normally appears as a localised painful swelling on the gingiva next to the tooth associated with the deep pocketing. The abscess usually drains through the pocket. A true pocket is formed once the periodontal disease destroys the periodontal membrane and the bone supporting the teeth.

6

Caries

1 When a cavity occurs, there have been various components that have aided cavitation. What needs to be present for caries to occur?
   A A tooth and sugar
   B Bacterial plaque and a tooth
   C Bacterial plaque, refined carbohydrate, a tooth, and time
   D Calculus, poor oral hygiene techniques, and erosion
   E Refined carbohydrates, a tooth, and gingival recession

2 Caries can occur on any surface of the tooth, but due to the structural shape of the tooth, there are certain areas that are easily cavitated. From the following options, which surfaces are most susceptible to caries?
   A Buccal and distal surfaces
   B Lingual and buccal surfaces
   C Lingual and occlusal surfaces
   D Occlusal surfaces and contact areas between adjacent teeth
   E Occlusal and buccal surfaces

3 In the mouth, remineralisation and demineralisation can occur multiple times during the day. What is meant by the term demineralisation?
   A When the enamel and dentine are exposed, and acidic ions leave the enamel of the tooth
   B When the enamel of the tooth softens due to high fruit juice consumption
   C When the pH balance falls below 5.5 pH and acidic ions leave the enamel of the tooth
   D When the pH balance goes higher than 5.5 pH and acidic ions leave the enamel of the tooth
   E When the teeth aren't brushed with fluoride toothpaste for long periods of time.

Questions and Answers in Oral Health Education, First Edition. Chloe Foxhall and Anna Lown.
© 2021 John Wiley & Sons Ltd. Published 2021 by John Wiley & Sons Ltd.
Companion website: www.wiley.com/go/foxhall/oral-health-education

4 In the mouth, remineralisation and demineralisation can occur multiple times during the day. What is meant by the term remineralisation?

A When the enamel of the tooth softens due to high fruit juice consumption

B When the pH balance of the mouth drops and acid attacks the enamel

C When the pH balance of the mouth rises back up to a safe level

D When the pH balance of the mouth rises back up to a safe level and saliva helps to return the calcium and phosphate ions to the enamel surface

E When the pH balance of the mouth rises back up to a safe level and saliva helps to return the calcium to the enamel surface

5 What is the ionic seesaw?

A The movement of calcium and phosphate ions going in and out of the dentine

B The movement of calcium and phosphate ions going in and out of the enamel

C The movement of fluoride and calcium during the change in the cell structure

D The movement of ions between the enamel and dentine

E The movement of phosphates around the oral cavity

6 After a period of time with frequent consumption of sugars, phosphates and calcium will be removed from the enamel. What is this process known as?

A Brown spot

B Demineralisation

C Fluorosis

D Remineralisation

E White spot

7 Miss Smith has a high caries rate and requires some advice from the oral health educator. What does the oral health educator suggest as being the most effective way of controlling the number of dental caries in the patient's mouth?

A Interdental cleaning

B Regular toothbrushing

C Reduce the frequency of sugar intake

D To eat the same snacks but just spread out throughout the day

E Use of fluoride mouthwash

8 What does DMF stand for?

A Decayed, missing, filled

B Decayed, missing, furcations

C Deciduous, missing, filled

D Displaced, missing, fillings

E Decayed, molar, fillings

9 A patient attends with their parents for an oral health session; after completing a diet sheet you notice that the patient is having regular snacks throughout the day. What advice from the options below would you give concerning the frequency of and the best time for snacks to be consumed?

A 4–5 times per day

B At meal times only

C As often as they would like

D Before brushing their teeth

E For breakfast

Extended Matching Questions

For each of the following questions, select the most appropriate answer from the list below. The answers might be used once, more than once or not at all.

Topic: Caries

a) Almost immediately
b) Clostridia
c) Fluorosis
d) Root caries
e) Spirochetes
f) Start of a cavity
g) Three hours
h) Xerostomia

1 When caries occur, there must be three bacteria present for this to happen. There is an acidogenic group that contains Streptococcus mutans and lactobacillus and a proteolytic group. Which of the answers is most suitable for the other bacteria required for caries to occur?

2 A Stephan's curve shows the demineralisation and remineralisation of a patient's mouth before, during, and after an acid attack. If acidic food is consumed, the pH level drops to a critical level. Which of the answers is most appropriate for how long it takes for the pH level to drop?

3 A 6-year-old male patient attended the dental practice for an exam appointment. During the examination, the dentist diagnoses a white spot lesion on the surface of the enamel. Which of the answers is most appropriate to explain the diagnosis?

Answers

1   When a cavity occurs, there have been various components that have aided cavitation. What needs to be present for caries to occur?

   Correct Answer: c) Bacterial plaque, refined carbohydrate, a tooth, and time

   In order for caries to occur, there must be a tooth, bacterial plaque (fermentable carbohydrate, which is the food source for plaque bacteria) and time.

2   Caries can occur on any surface of the tooth, but due to the structural shape of the tooth, there are certain areas that are easily cavitated. From the following options, which surfaces are most susceptible to caries?

   Correct Answer: d) Occlusal surfaces and contact areas between adjacent teeth

   Common sites for caries to occur would be occlusal surfaces, particularly newly erupted molars and premolars, in the pits and fissures of the teeth and contact areas between adjacent teeth. Other common sites could be cervical margins near to the gingival margin, root surfaces, molar teeth on the buccal surfaces, and palatal grooves on the upper anterior teeth.

3   In the mouth, remineralisation and demineralisation can occur multiple times during the day. What is meant by the term demineralisation?

   Correct Answer: c) When the pH balance falls below 5.5 pH and acidic ions leave the enamel of the tooth

   When the pH balance falls below the neutral pH of 5.5, the teeth go into a critical stage. During this acidic change, calcium and phosphate ions leave the enamel of the tooth which in turn makes the enamel much softer. If demineralisation occurs more frequently than remineralisation, then this is when caries will occur. The Stephan's curve demonstrates the cariogenic challenge of a tooth.

4   In the mouth, remineralisation and demineralisation can occur multiple times during the day. What is meant by the term remineralisation?

   Correct Answer: d) When the pH balance of the mouth rises back up to a safe level and saliva helps to return the calcium and phosphate ions to the enamel surface

   Remineralisation is when the saliva acts as a neutraliser to help neutralise the plaque acids within the oral cavity. Saliva contains bicarbonate ions that help return the calcium and phosphate ions to the enamel surfaces of the teeth. This process is called the buffer action. The remineralisation of the oral cavity can take between 30 minutes and 2 hours for the pH balance to return back to a safe level.

5 What is the ionic seesaw?

Correct Answer: b) The movement of calcium and phosphate ions going in and out of the enamel

The ionic seesaw relates to a theory produced in 1977 by Levine. The theory relates to a chemical relationship between enamel plaque and factors that determine the movement of calcium and phosphate ions from saliva/plaque to enamel and vice versa.

6 After a period of time with frequent consumption of sugars, phosphates and calcium will be removed from the enamel. What is this process known as?

Correct Answer: d) Demineralisation

Demineralisation is when the pH balance falls below the neutral pH of 5.5 and the teeth go into a critical stage. During this acidic change, calcium and phosphate ions leave the enamel of the tooth which in turn makes the enamel much softer. If demineralisation occurs more frequently than remineralisation, this is when caries will occur. Stephan's curve demonstrates the cariogenic challenge of a tooth.

7 Miss Smith has a high caries rate and requires some advice from the oral health educator. What does the oral health educator suggest as being the most effective way of controlling the amount of dental caries in the patient's mouth?

Correct Answer: c) Reduce the frequency of sugar intake

In order for caries to occur, there must be a high frequency of sugar intake. Limiting the frequency of sugar intake will help to eliminate the constant demineralisation and remineralisation cycle and help to minimise the cariogenic challenge of a tooth.

8 What does DMF stand for?

Correct Answer: a) Decayed, missing, filled

The DMFT index is a quantitative expression of an individual's lifetime disease experience. It stands for Decayed Missing Filled and can be used in either permanent or deciduous dentition. If used in deciduous dentition, the expression would be written in lowercase letters: dmft.

9 A patient attends with their parents for an oral health session; after completing a diet sheet you notice that the patient is having regular snacks throughout the day. What advice from the options below would you give concerning the frequency of and the best time for snacks to be consumed?

Correct Answer: b) At meal times only

If a patient likes to eat sweets and chocolates, and would prefer not to stop eating them entirely, then it is best to eat them at mealtimes only. Eating them at mealtimes only helps to reduce the frequency of sugary foods being eaten during the day and should therefore help to prevent the occurrence of caries.

Extended Matching Questions

Topic: Caries

1 When caries occur there must be three bacteria present for this to happen. There is an acidogenic group that contains *Streptococcus mutans* and lactobacillus and a proteolytic group. Which of the answers is most suitable for the other bacteria required for caries to occur?

Correct Answer: b) Clostridia

For caries to occur, three bacteria's must be present. Clostridia is in the proteolytic group; these bacteria dissolve the proteins. *Streptococcus mutans* and lactobacillus are in the acidogenic group; these produce acid and remove mineral salts. The acidogenic group removes mineral salts first. When the caries reach the dentine, the proteolytic group begins to act by dissolving proteins.

2 A Stephan's curve shows the demineralisation and remineralisation of a patient's mouth before, during, and after an acid attack. If acidic food is consumed, the pH level drops to a critical level. Which of the answers is most appropriate for how long it takes for the pH level to drop?

Correct Answer: a) Almost immediately

The pH level of the mouth can drop to critical in 2 minutes or less during an acid attack. It can take between 30 minutes and 2 hours to rise back to a safe level. Frequent intake of sugar will allow the pH level to remain at a critical level for a lot longer, which is when caries can occur.

3 A 6-year-old male patient attended the dental practice for an exam appointment. During the examination, the dentist diagnoses a white spot lesion on the surface of the enamel. Which of the answers is most appropriate to explain the diagnosis?

Correct Answer: f) Start of a cavity

The early stages of a cavity show as a white spot on the surface of the enamel. The spot becomes rough and can become stained if present for a while. This stage is much easier to see on the smooth surfaces of the teeth, unlike fissures. If the lesion progresses, the surface of the enamel disintegrates and a cavity forms.

7

Sugar

1 Eating sugar can be part of a balanced diet; however, non-milk extrinsic sugars should be avoided. What kinds of food would you find these in?
   A Cakes, biscuits, and chocolate
   B Dairy products
   C Fruit, vegetables, and seeds
   D Meat
   E Rice, pasta, and bread

2 Which of the following sugars is non-milk extrinsic (free sugars)?
   A Lactitol
   B Lactose
   C Mannitol
   D Sucrose
   E Xylitol

3 Sugars are separated into groups to help differentiate between the different types. Which organisation first introduced the classification for sugars?
   A COMA – Committee on Medical Aspects
   B MAFF – Ministry of Agriculture, Fisheries, and Foods
   C NEBDN – National Examination Board for Dental Nurses
   D SACN – Scientific Advisory Committee on Nutrition
   E WHO – World Health Organisation

4 A patient's diet sheet shows that the majority of the snacks being consumed are intrinsic sugars. From the following options, which food or drink contains intrinsic sugars?
   A A bowl of cereal with semi-skimmed milk
   B A chicken pie
   C A fresh fruit salad
   D Chocolate cake
   E Ginger nut cookie

Questions and Answers in Oral Health Education, First Edition. Chloe Foxhall and Anna Lown.
© 2021 John Wiley & Sons Ltd. Published 2021 by John Wiley & Sons Ltd.
Companion website: www.wiley.com/go/foxhall/oral-health-education

5   Often, patients will tell you they have replaced sugar in baking or in hot drinks with a sweetener option. Sweeteners are suggested as an alternative to help patients reduce their sugar intake but it is generally consider better to remove as many sweet tasting foods and drinks as possible from a diet. Which of the following answers supports this?

    A Patients who eat food with sugar in are at less risk of decay than patients who eat food with sweeteners

    B Patients who have sugar free medications are at higher risk of caries when eating sweeteners.

    C Sweeteners are put into food to mask the amount of sugar in the food

    D Sweeteners cause decay in deciduous teeth

    E Sweeteners do not cause caries, but they do encourage a sweet tooth.

6   A parent attends the dental practice for some advice on diet for their 6-year-old son who will only eat a chocolate breakfast cereal with five teaspoons of sugar. Which piece of advice out of the following would you give the parent?

    A It doesn't matter what the child eats for breakfast; he is too young to remember what he eats every morning

    B The child is better off eating breakfast as he likes it, then brushing his teeth

    C The child should be allowed to decide what he wants to eat for breakfast

    D The child should carry on eating the chocolate breakfast cereal as long as he stops having spoonful's of sugar on top

    E The child should change his breakfast to something without sugar to prevent caries forming.

7   The Committee on Medical Aspects (COMA) is closely connected with the oral health advice that we provide. Which of the following statements is true?

    A A COMA report recommends that dental professionals should advise patients to do their own research on oral health advice to save clinician time

    B A COMA report recommends that elderly people with their teeth should restrict the frequency of non-milk extrinsic sugars because of the decrease in saliva flow means they may be more at risk of caries

    C A COMA report recommends that providing food for communities should allow for everyone to have a portion of non-milk extrinsic sugar so no one is missing out

    D A COMA report recommends that schools should supply desserts that contain non-milk extrinsic sugars at lunch times to make children excited about attending school

    E A COMA report recommends that to get a baby or toddler to hold a dummy or bottle in their mouth, it can be coated in jam or sugar.

Extended Matching Questions

For each of the following questions, select the most appropriate answer from the list below. The answers might be used once, more than once, or not at all.

a) Caries
b) Confectionary
c) Milk sugars
d) Non-milk extrinsics
e) Reduced saliva flow
f) Raw vegetables
g) Talking
h) Water

1   A mum attends a dental practice to discuss diet advice for her three children; their ages vary between 3 and 8. All children eat a balanced diet apart from the cookies they eat in the evening for dessert. Which of the options would you suggest the mum gives the children after the cookies?

2   A school chef is trying to decide on a snack for a school menu and contacts you to ask what snacks he could offer children that don't contain sugars that could cause caries. Which of the above would you advise?

3   An elderly lady visits the dental practice for her check-up. During the appointment the dentist notices she has multiple root caries. He briefly discusses her diet with her, which reveals the patient has a healthy diet apart from hard-boiled sweets which she eats in the evening. Which of the above would be a contributing factor to the root caries along with the already consumed non-milk extrinsic sugars?

Answers

1 Eating sugar can be part of a balanced diet; however, non-milk extrinsic sugars should be avoided. What kinds of food would you find these in?

Correct Answer: a) Cakes, biscuits, and chocolate.

Non-milk extrinsic are bad sugars that are harmful to your teeth and can be cariogenic. Another sugar group is intrinsic sugars which are found in whole (raw) fruit and vegetables. The sugar is part of the cell found in foods and the reason these do not cause caries is because they are broken down and digested in the stomach. The final sugar group is milk sugars, which are naturally found in milk and milk products. Sugar occurs naturally in milk and is also digested in the stomach.

2 Which of the following sugars is non-milk extrinsic (free sugars)?

Correct Answer: d) Sucrose

Sucrose is the main sugar found in these types of food. Other examples of sugars are fructose and glucose.

3 Sugars are separated into groups to help differentiate between the different types. Which organisation first introduced the classification for sugars?

Correct Answer: a) COMA – Committee on Medical Aspects

COMA introduced the classifications for sugars.

4 A patient's diet sheet shows that the majority of the snacks being consumed are intrinsic sugars. From the following options, which food or drink contains intrinsic sugars?

Correct Answer: c) A fresh fruit salad

Fruit and vegetables contain intrinsic sugars. As soon as the cell structure changes (i.e. cooking), the intrinsic sugars become non-milk extrinsics as they are digested in the mouth – which can cause decay.

5 Often, patients will tell you they have replaced sugar in baking or in hot drinks with a sweetener option. Sweeteners are suggested as an alternative to help patients reduce their sugar intake but it is generally consider better to remove as many sweet tasting foods and drinks as possible from a diet. Which of the following answers supports this?

Correct Answer: e) Sweeteners do not cause caries, but they do encourage a sweet tooth

Artificial sweeteners come in two different categories: bulk and intense. Some of the common sweetener names are: Mannitol, Sorbitol, and hydrogenated glucose syrup. Artificial sweeteners are non-cariogenic, although some do have a mild laxative effect.

6 A parent attends the dental practice for some advice on diet for their 6-year-old son who will only eat a chocolate breakfast cereal with five teaspoons of sugar. Which piece of advice out of the following would you give the parent?

Correct Answer: e) The child should change his breakfast to something without sugar to prevent caries forming

In an ideal situation, the child should have an alternative breakfast to something containing sugar. A meal plan should be looked at to include fresh fruit and a healthier option; for example, porridge.

7 The Committee on Medical Aspects (COMA) is closely connected with the oral health advice that we provide. Which of the following statements is true?

Correct Answer: b) A COMA report recommended that elderly people with their teeth should restrict the frequency of non-milk extrinsic sugars because their decrease in saliva flow means they may be more at risk of caries

If someone has a decreased saliva flow (xerostomia) then they are more at risk of dental disease. If there is less saliva flow in the oral cavity, then there is less saliva to neutralise the dietary acids, leading to dental caries.

Extended Matching Questions

1 A mum attends a dental practice to discuss diet advice for her three children; their ages vary between 3 and 8. All children eat a balanced diet apart from the cookies they eat in the evening for dessert. Which of the options would you suggest the mum gives the children after the cookies?

Correct Answer: h) Water

Water and milk are classed as safer options of drink to consume. Having water after a meal will help to dislodge any food debris that may be present in the fissures of the posterior teeth. This then cuts down the contact time with the non-milk extrinsic sugar and the tooth, which in turn will help to prevent caries formation. This action is called the buffer action.

2 A school chef is trying to decide on a snack for a school menu and contacts you to ask what snacks he could offer children that don't contain sugars that could cause caries. Which of the above would you advise?

Correct Answer: f) Raw vegetables

Having raw vegetables for a snack is an extremely healthy option. The sugars present in the raw vegetables are intrinsic and are therefore not harmful to the teeth, as the vegetables are in their original, raw form.

3   An elderly lady visits the dental practice for her check-up. During the appointment, the dentist notices she has multiple root caries. He briefly discusses her diet with her, which reveals the patient has a healthy diet apart from hard-boiled sweets which she eats in the evening. Which of the above would be a contributing factor to the root caries along with the already consumed non-milk extrinsic sugars?

Correct Answer: e) Reduced saliva flow

Elderly patients more often suffer from a degree of decreased saliva flow. This, combined with the consumption of non-milk extrinsic sugars, is going to put the patient at more risk of caries formation. Root caries spread more rapidly than caries on the enamel surface, as the root of the tooth does not contain enamel and caries spread much quicker through the cementum and then into the dentine.

8

Tooth Surface Loss

1 A 35-year-old female attends the dental practice for her routine dental exam appointment. The patient complains of sensitivity. The dentist confirms tooth surface wear and faceting on the anterior teeth, upper and lower. Which of the following is the correct term for this tooth surface loss?

A Abfraction
B Abrasion
C Attrition
D Caries
E Erosion

2 A 50-year-old female attends the dental practice for her routine dental exam appointment. The patient has no complaints. The dentist diagnoses surface loss on the labial surfaces. Which of the following is the correct term for this tooth surface loss?

A Abfraction
B Abrasion
C Attrition
D Caries
E Erosion

3 A 68-year-old female attends the dental practice for her routine dental exam appointment. The patient has no complaints. The dentist diagnoses surface loss along the cervical margin. Which of the following is the correct term for this tooth surface loss?

A Abfraction
B Abrasion
C Attrition
D Caries
E Erosion

Questions and Answers in Oral Health Education, First Edition. Chloe Foxhall and Anna Lown.
© 2021 John Wiley & Sons Ltd. Published 2021 by John Wiley & Sons Ltd.
Companion website: www.wiley.com/go/foxhall/oral-health-education

4 Non-carious tooth surface loss can occur as a result of a patient's habits or normal wear and tear. Select the most likely cause of dental erosion from the list below.
   A Brushing teeth too vigorously
   B Leaving dentures in chemical solutions overnight
   C Poor oral hygiene
   D The effects of gastric reflux acids on teeth
   E The frequent intake of sugary snacks and drinks

5 You are talking with a colleague about dental erosion; which of the following options consists of two contributing factors of dental erosion?
   A Gastric reflux and caries
   B Gastric reflux and fizzy drinks
   C Medication and plaque
   D Plaque and caries
   E Plaque and water

6 Erosion doesn't affect every patient that enters a dental surgery; there can be a range of different causes. Which type of patient may be more likely to present with erosion from the options below?
   A A patient with a healthy diet who only drinks water and milk
   B A patient who eats a lot of chocolate and cakes
   C A patient who plays a lot of sports and drinks a lot of energy drinks
   D A patient who drinks fizzy once per day and has a healthy diet otherwise
   E A patient who eats sweets once a week

7 Abfraction is another type of tooth surface loss. From the options below, what best describes abfraction?
   A Mechanical non-carious tooth surface loss of the buccal surface
   B Mechanical non-carious tooth surface loss of the gingival margin
   C Non-carious tooth surface loss of the fissures
   D Non-carious tooth surface loss of the occlusal surfaces
   E Non-carious tooth surface loss of the palatal surface.

8 A patient has attended the dental surgery for an assessment appointment. The dentist diagnoses abrasion around the cervical margins on the canines. From the options listed, what option explains how abrasion can happen?
   A Eating sweets throughout the day
   B Hard toothbrushing
   C Soft toothbrushing
   D Too many fizzy drinks
   E Too many fruit juices

Extended Matching Questions

For each of the following questions, select the most appropriate answer from the list below. The answers might be used once, more than once, or not at all.

Topic: Tooth Surface loss

a) Abfraction
b) Abrasion
c) Anorexia
d) Attrition
e) Bulimia
f) Bruxism
g) Excessive toothbrushing
h) Faceting

1   Tooth surface loss due to recurring acid attack can affect the occlusal surfaces on the lower molars and the palatal or labial surfaces on the upper anteriors. From the answers listed, please select the most appropriate answer that can cause this.

2   When giving toothbrushing instructions for a patient, you are demonstrating the scrub technique and you tell the patient to only apply gentle pressure while cleaning. From the answers listed, please select the most appropriate reason for what tooth surface loss you are trying to avoid.

Answers

1 A 35-year-old female attends the dental practice for their routine dental exam appointment. The patient complains of sensitivity. The dentist confirms tooth surface wear and faceting on the anterior teeth, upper and lower on the incisal surfaces. Which of the following is the correct term for this tooth surface loss?

Correct Answer: c) Attrition

Attrition is caused by bruxism, which is usually a subconscious habit. Attrition would be found on the incisal or occlusal surfaces of the teeth. The action of clenching or grinding wears at the enamel, creating facets which can eventually go through to the dentine. Caries is caused by refined sugar and bacterial plaque after a period of time. Erosion is surface loss, usually on the palatal and labial surfaces due to acid attack. Abfraction is surface loss caused by tooth fracture, usually affecting cervical areas of heavily loaded teeth. Abrasion is surface loss caused by vigorous toothbrushing, usually along the cervical margin.

2 A 50-year-old female attends the dental practice for her routine dental exam appointment. The patient has no complaints. The dentist diagnoses surface loss on the labial surfaces. Which of the following is the correct term for this tooth surface loss?

Correct Answer: e) Erosion

Erosion is surface loss, usually on the palatal and labial surfaces due to acid attack. The acid wears away at the enamel, causing pits on the labial or palatal surfaces. This is commonly caused by food or drink with a strong concentration of acidic properties, such as fruit juice. Abrasion is surface loss caused by vigorous toothbrushing, usually along the cervical margin. Abfraction is surface loss caused by tooth fracture, usually affecting cervical areas of heavily loaded teeth. Attrition is wear at the enamel creating facets on the incisal or occlusal surfaces.

3 A 68-year-old female attends the dental practice for her routine dental exam appointment. The patient has no complaints. The dentist diagnoses surface loss along the cervical margin. Which of the following is the correct term for this tooth surface loss?

Correct Answer: b) Abrasion

Abrasion is surface loss caused by vigorous toothbrushing, usually along the cervical margin. It is common to cause abrasion on the canines and the premolars as they are usually the most protruding. Lesions are usually more wide than they are deep; however, if the tooth brushing technique is not changed, they can become deep and become sensitive. Erosion is surface loss, usually on the palatal and labial surfaces due to acid attack. Abfraction is surface loss caused by tooth fracture, usually affecting cervical areas of heavily loaded teeth. Attrition is wear at the enamel creating facets on the incisal or occlusal surfaces.

4 Non-carious tooth surface loss can occur as a result of a patient's habits or normal wear and tear. Select the most likely cause of dental erosion from the list below.

Correct Answer: d) The effects of gastric reflux acids on teeth

The acid present in vomit is extremely acidic and can cause dental erosion. If a patient was to suffer from gastric reflux, then the acid produced from the stomach and into the oral cavity would cause erosion of the dentition.

5 You are talking with a colleague about dental erosion; which of the following options consists of two contributing factors of dental erosion?

Correct Answer: b) Gastric reflux and fizzy drinks

Irreversible tooth surface loss is due to a chemical dissolution by acids that are not of bacterial origin. It is mostly seen on the occlusal, palatal, and lingual surfaces of the teeth. It is mainly due to dietary acids; for example, fruit juice and fizzy drinks. Medication can be a risk, especially if it is recreational, as can lifestyle habits; for example, holding fizzy drinks in the mouth or constantly sipping fizzy drinks or fruit juice.

6 Erosion doesn't affect every patient that enters a dental surgery; there can be a range of different causes. Which type of patient may be more likely to present with erosion from the options below?

Correct Answer: c) A patient who plays a lot of sports and drinks a lot of energy drinks

Energy drinks have a lot of sugar and acid in them and can cause erosion of the dentition. If a sports player is constantly drinking these acidic drinks, then this can cause erosion. These drinks are often sipped as opposed to being drunk in one go.

7 Abfraction is another type of tooth surface loss. From the options below, what best describes abfraction?

Correct Answer: b) Mechanical non-carious tooth surface loss of the gingival margin

Abfraction is a form of non-carious tooth tissue loss that occurs along the gingival margin. It is a mechanical loss of tooth structure that is not caused by tooth decay. These lesions occur in both the dentine and enamel of the tooth.

8 A patient has attended the dental surgery for an assessment appointment. The dentist diagnoses abrasion around the cervical margins on the canines. From the options listed, what option explains how abrasion can happen?

Correct Answer: b) Hard toothbrushing

Abrasion can happen due to mechanical factors such as toothbrush abrasion, oral or facial piercings, and habits like biting pens, etc.

Extended Matching Questions

For each of the following questions, select the most appropriate answer from the list below. The answers might be used once, more than once, or not at all.

Topic: Tooth surface loss

1   Tooth surface loss due to recurring acid attack can affect the occlusal surfaces on the lower molars and the palatal or labial surfaces on the upper anteriors. From the answers listed, please select the most appropriate answer that can cause this.
    Correct Answer: e) Bulimia

    Bulimia is an emotional disorder usually characterised by a person wanting to lose weight and often going to extreme measures, such as self-induced vomiting. Vomiting can bring a lot of acid into the mouth, which can cause tooth surface loss on the occlusal surfaces of the lower molars and the palatal or labial surfaces.

2   When giving toothbrushing instructions for a patient, you are demonstrating the scrub technique and you tell the patient to only apply gentle pressure while cleaning. From the answers listed, please select the most appropriate reason for what tooth surface loss you are trying to avoid.
    Correct Answer: b) Abrasion

    Tooth brushing too vigorously can cause surface loss at the cervical margin, also known as abrasion. It is best to teach patients to be gentle from a young age to avoid this in the future. The evidence of vigorous toothbrushing is often not visible for many years.

9

Visual Aids

1   The ERI is used to assess readability, jargon, layout, range of topics covered, and interest. What does ERI stand for?
    A Ease of range interest
    B Ease of reading index
    C Easy reading information
    D Easy readability index
    E Ease of red information

2   SMOG is used as a measurement when assessing literature that may be provided to patients. What does SMOG stand for?
    A Select measuring of grounding text
    B Simple measure of gobbledygook
    C Simple measurement of good information
    D Simplified measurement of gobbledygook
    E Sound measure of gobbledygook

3   When speaking to patients, it can be easy for you to use jargon in your explanations; this can prevent the patient from learning. What is the main reason we avoid using jargon when delivering oral health messages?
    A To confuse the patient
    B To help the patient understand what we are talking about
    C To make sure the patient knows we are qualified in this subject
    D To sound Intelligent
    E To sound smart

Questions and Answers in Oral Health Education, First Edition. Chloe Foxhall and Anna Lown.
© 2021 John Wiley & Sons Ltd. Published 2021 by John Wiley & Sons Ltd.
Companion website: www.wiley.com/go/foxhall/oral-health-education

4   Visual aids hold a lot of advantages when providing oral health sessions. From the following options, which is a disadvantage to visual aids?

A Can make the lesson more interesting

B Helps the students learn

C Helps to make the student more alert

D If teaching on a one to one basis then it gives the student something to look at other that the educator

E Leaflets and posters produced by manufacturers are often advertising something

5   A student attends an oral health session but struggles to concentrate for long periods of time and is a kinaesthetic learner. At the next session, what visual aid would you use from the following?

A A jigsaw

B A video

C A worksheet

D Demonstration models

E Story pictures

Extended Matching Questions

For each of the following questions, select the most appropriate answer from the list below. The answers might be used once, more than once, or not at all.

Topic: Visual aids

a) Age index

b) Creates interest

c) Expense

d) Helps the student learn

e) Jargon

f) SMOG index

g) Student alertness

h) The memory can remember what it has seen more than what it has heard

1   You and another oral health educator are preparing for a session with multiple learners. You are discussing resources and you bring up that you would like to use food packets as a visual aid. Which of the answers is the most appropriate for a disadvantage for visual aids?

2   You are creating a leaflet for patients based around orthodontic appliance care. You have finished the leaflet and are checking the ease of reading index (ERI) to ensure that the reading age is appropriate for the person who will receive the leaflet. Which of the answers is the most appropriate way to test the ERI?

Answers

1   The ERI is used to assess readability, jargon, layout, range of topics covered, and interest. What does ERI stand for?

Correct Answer: b) Ease of reading index

The ease of reading index is used to ensure the literature given to students is suitable for them. It covers readability, jargon, layout, range of topics covered, and interest.

2   SMOG is used as a measurement when assessing literature that may be providing patients. What does SMOG stand for?

Correct Answer: b) Simple measure of gobbledygook

The SMOG index is a measurement to show the readability level of a piece of literature to assess which target group it would be suitable for.

3   When speaking to patients, it can be easy for you to use jargon in your explanations; this can prevent the patient from learning. What is the main reason we avoid using jargon when delivering oral health messages?

Correct Answer: b) To help the patient understand what we are talking about

During a session you should try to avoid using jargon when talking to patients to prevent them from getting confused. Through using simple terminology, the patient should understand the information you are providing, which should then be retained and implemented.

4   Visual aids hold a lot of advantages when providing oral health sessions. From the following options, which is a disadvantage to visual aids?

Correct Answer: e) Leaflets and posters produced by manufacturers are often advertising something

Visual aids can be a great way to help patients learn, they can be used for all ages and can be very educational, but some visual aids can have a disadvantage as they are often advertising a product or company. Other disadvantages can be that they are expensive and if they are overhandled they can be damaged or broken.

5   A student attends an oral health session but struggles to concentrate for long periods of time and is a kinaesthetic learner. At the next session, what visual aid would you use from the following?

Correct Answer: d) Demonstration models

A kinaesthetic learner will take more information away when they are shown physically how to do something. Using a demonstration model is a good way to incorporate this into an oral hygiene session.

Extended Matching Questions

Topic: Visual aids

1 You and another oral health educator are preparing for a session with multiple learners. You are discussing resources and you bring up that you would like to use food packets as a visual aid. Which of the answers is the most appropriate for a disadvantage for visual aids?

Correct Answer: c) Expense

Using visual aids can be a great way to help the students learn. It can make the students more alert and the memory can often retain what it has seen more than what it has heard. A disadvantage to visual aids is that they come at an expense; it is hard to gain visual aids that you have not had to pay for, so when you are first starting this has to be considered.

2 You are creating a leaflet for patients based around orthodontic appliance care. You have finished the leaflet and are checking the ease of reading index (ERI) to ensure that the reading age is appropriate for the person who will receive the leaflet. Which of the answers is the most appropriate way to test the ERI?

Correct Answer: f) SMOG index

SMOG is the acronym derived from simple measure of gobbledygook. This is completed the following steps:

1) Select text.
2) Count 10 sentences.
3) Count up all the words with 3 or more syllables.
4) Multiply your answer by 3.
5) Find the number closest to your answer from the following: 1 4 9 16 25 36 49 64 81 100 121 144 169
6) Find the square root of the number you have circled (1–1 4–2 9–3 16–4 25–5 36–6, etc.).
7) Add 8.
8) Readability level =

Once you have worked out the SMOG index, the readability level is the minimum age of who can receive the document.

10

Aims and Objectives

1 When planning an oral health session, you should also set out aims, objectives, and learning outcomes. What phrase would you find in the aim of an oral health session?
   A During the session the learner will be able demonstrate where the sugars are stated on a food packet
   B During this session the learner will develop a better understanding of hidden sugars in food and drink
   C During the session the learner will be able to state the causes of caries
   D The learning outcome of the session is that the learner will be able to pick out foods with hidden sugars
   E The learning outcome of the session is that the learner will be able to state the cause of caries

2 When planning an oral health session, you should also set out aims, objectives, and learning outcomes. From the following options, which one best describes the use of an objective?
   A A guide for the course provider
   B A guide to the learner
   C A guide to a teacher
   D An objective is what the learner will be able to do by the end of the session
   E Another name for a lesson plan

3 You have been asked to create a lesson plan for a 2 hour session that will have 10 learners; you have already chosen your topic. Which of the following options should be included to record how you propose to deliver the session?
   A Break time
   B Fire exits
   C Room layout
   D Teaching methods
   E Teacher's qualifications

Questions and Answers in Oral Health Education, First Edition. Chloe Foxhall and Anna Lown.
© 2021 John Wiley & Sons Ltd. Published 2021 by John Wiley & Sons Ltd.
Companion website: www.wiley.com/go/foxhall/oral-health-education

4 A lesson is usually split into three sections: a beginning, a middle, and an end. From the following options, select the most appropriate answer that explains what the beginning should include.

A The assessment

B The evaluation

C The feedback for the lesson

D The session summary

E What you expect learners to learn during the session

5 During a lesson you are planning, you add in time for the learners to have a discussion. What are the advantages to this?

A Breaks up the session

B It can cause learners to become distracted

C Learners can share ideas and then copy each other's answers

D Spontaneous and gives the group shared knowledge

E Stops the lesson from being repetitive

6 When planning a lesson, you ensure you have the correct resources for that lesson; one of these resources could be an evaluation. From the following answers, which of the following best explains what an evaluation is?

A Evaluation is the overall feedback from the learners

B Evaluation is the overall feedback from the teacher

C Evaluation is the process by which the effects of the assessment can be determined

D Evaluation is the process by which the effects and effectiveness of teaching can be determined

E Evaluation is the process by which the learner can evaluate their own work

7 When planning an oral health session, you should set out aims, objectives, and learning outcomes. From the following options, which answer best explains what an aim is?

A An aim is a general statement that explains the evaluation process of the session being taught

B An aim is a general statement that explains what the learner will be able to do at the end of the session

C An aim is a general statement that explains what the teacher wants the learners to be able to do

D An aim is the guide for the teacher and learner to develop together after the session has been taught

E An aim is a guide to a teacher

8 You are planning a lesson based around diet for a group of pre-school children's parents; what assessment method will you use to best test your objectives?

A Demonstration

B Discussion

C Game

D Practical

E Role play

Extended Matching Questions

For each of the following questions, select the most appropriate answer from the list below. The answers might be used once, more than once, or not at all.

Topic: Aims and Objectives

a) Aim
b) Description
c) Discussion
d) Lecture
e) Notes section
f) Objective
g) Subject
h) Teaching methods

1   You are planning a lesson for a group of school children; you are creating the lesson plan and you have written 'during this session the students will develop a better understanding of hidden sugars in foods'. Which of the answers is the most appropriate for what you have written?

2   You are planning a lesson for a group of school children; you are creating a lesson plan and you have written 'identify which foods contain hidden sugars'. Which of the answers is the most appropriate for what you have written?

3   You have almost finished making your lesson plans for a day of visiting different classes in a junior school. You have included the subject, aims, objectives, and the details about the students and the school. Which of the answers is most appropriate for something you should include in a lesson plan?

4   You are holding a session with five children regarding hidden sugars in food; you gather the children around a table in a circle. You start talking about the foods you eat which contain sugar, inviting the children to join in. Which of the answers is the most appropriate for the teaching method you are trying to use?

Answers

1   When planning an oral health session, you should also set out aims, objectives, and learning outcomes. What phrase would you find in the aim of an oral health session?

Correct Answer: b) During this session the learners will develop a better understanding of hidden sugars in food and drink.

An aim is a guide for the teacher and should be able to give the learners an idea of what will be expected of them during that session.

2   When planning an oral health session, you should also set out aims, objectives, and learning outcomes. From the following options, which one best describes the use of an objective?

Correct Answer: d) An objective is what the learner will be able to do by the end of the session

An objective is measurable and should always contain a doing word. This gives the learners an idea of what they should be learning throughout this session.

3   You have been asked to create a lesson plan for a 2 hour session that will have 10 learners; you have already chosen your topic. Which of the following options should be included to record how you propose to deliver the session?

Correct Answer: d) Teaching methods

A lesson plan should tell you what you are teaching, when and where you are teaching, how many learners you have and the aims and objectives, and teaching methods of the lesson.

4   A lesson is usually split up into three sections: a beginning, a middle, and an end. From the following options, select the most appropriate answer that explains what the beginning should include?

Correct Answer: e) What you expect learners to learn during the session

The beginning of a lesson should be a brief introduction to yourself and the lesson, outlining the aims and objectives. The middle of the lesson should be where the new information is provided and the end of the lesson should test the objectives and a conclusion of the lesson.

5   During a lesson you are planning, you should add in time for the learners to have a discussion. What are the advantages to this?

Correct Answer: d) Spontaneous and gives the group shared knowledge

Discussion during a lesson can allow learners time to share ideas and thoughts, which can lead to further learning. Discussion can also form good working relationships for learners to express views on the subject matter.

6 When planning a lesson, you ensure you have the correct resources for that lesson; one of these resources could be an evaluation. From the following answers, which of the following best explains what an evaluation is?

Correct Answer: d) Evaluation is the process by which the effects and effectiveness of teaching can be determined.

An evaluation of the lesson can be done verbally, in the form of questions and answers or as an assignment sent home with the learners. Completing an evaluation at the end of each lesson can give the teacher a better understanding of what the learner has understood and where they can start the next lesson.

7 When planning an oral health session, you should set out aims, objectives, and learning outcomes. From the following options, which answer best explains what an aim is?

Correct Answer: c) An aim is a general statement that explains what the teacher wants the learners to be able to do

An aim is provided by the teacher for each lesson and is what the teacher is planning to complete throughout the lesson.

8 You are planning a lesson based around diet for a group of pre-school children's parents; what assessment method will you use to best test your objectives?

Correct Answer: b) Discussion

A discussion would be the most preferred method of testing the knowledge of the children's parents. You could use written questions and answers; however, these may not be received well as the parents may feel that they are being formally tested. A discussion around the topic being taught would be sufficient to meet the needs of the parents and would be good to share ideas and knowledge.

Extended Matching Questions

Topic: Aims and Objectives

1 You are planning a lesson for a group of school children; you are creating a lesson plan and you have written 'during this session the students will develop a better understanding of hidden sugars in foods'. Which of the answers is the most appropriate for what you have written?

Correct Answer: a) Aim

An aim is put in place as a guide to the teacher; it consists of one, two, or three sentences that explain what you want the learners to be able to do. It is a statement that is not measurable on what is or can be achieved.

2 You are planning a lesson for a group of school children; you are creating a lesson plan and you have written 'identify which foods contain hidden sugars'. Which of the answers is the most appropriate for what you have written?

Correct Answer: f) Objective

An objective is put in place for the learners to be able to understand what they should achieve by the end of the session. The learning objective should also contain a doing word. The objective describes the terminal behaviour and is measured by time. Objectives should always start with the measurable part and should finish with what the task will be. Objectives should be SMART which stands for: Specific, Measurable, Attainable, Relevant, and Time related.

3 You have almost finished making your lesson plans for a day of visiting different classes in a junior school. You have included the subject, aims, objectives, and the details about the students and the school. Which of the answers is most appropriate for something you should include in a lesson plan?

Correct Answer: h) Teaching methods

Teaching methods should be included in a lesson plan to show that you are using a different range of methods to teach. Therefore, if you have a diverse group of learners you are able to get your aim across to the students through multiple methods.

4 You are holding a session with five children regarding hidden sugars in food; you gather the children around a table in a circle. You start talking about the foods you eat which contain sugar, inviting the children to join in. Which of the answers is the most appropriate for the teaching method you are trying to use?

Correct Answer: c) Discussion

A discussion is a group talk about a topic; it will be started and directed by the teacher to ensure the topic is continued throughout. The advantage of discussion is that it is spontaneous and allows the group to share knowledge – you may get information that you were not necessarily expecting. Students can learn from each other as well as the teacher. The disadvantages of discussion are that it is easy for learners to get sidetracked and some people can mishear information. You also may get a shy learner who doesn't feel comfortable participating.

11

Lesson Preparation and Communication

1 When planning a lesson, you have a lot of things to consider, such as target audience and the topic. From the following options, which are two considerations that need to be taken into account when setting an objective?
   A Objective needs to be appropriate to the target audience and suitable for the setting
   B Objective needs to be actioned at the end of the session along with the aim
   C Objective needs to be an activity taking place and state the resources being used
   D Objective needs to be based on gender and possible implications
   E Objective needs to be based on the correct topic and advised at the end of the lesson

2 An objective must be measured to show that the patient has learned. From the following options, how is an objective measured?
   A By how many attend
   B By the topic covered
   C By time
   D By the teacher's preference
   E By the venue

3 A lesson can be planned based on aims and objectives. SMART objectives were created to combine them with the learning outcomes. What does SMART stand for?
   A Smart, meaningful, attainable, realistic, and time bound
   B Smart, measurable, achievable, ready, and time
   C Specific, memorable, accurate, ready, and timely
   D Specific, measurable, accurate, realistic, and time bound
   E Specific, measurable, attainable, relevant, and time related

Questions and Answers in Oral Health Education, First Edition. Chloe Foxhall and Anna Lown.
© 2021 John Wiley & Sons Ltd. Published 2021 by John Wiley & Sons Ltd.
Companion website: www.wiley.com/go/foxhall/oral-health-education

4   You have been asked to plan a lesson for five patients; before you start creating the lesson plan, you have something to consider. Using the following options, what would you consider before starting the lesson plan?

   A Any electrical points and how many people will be in attendance
   B How many students there will be
   C How many students there will be and how big the venue is
   D How many students there will be, the venue, the time it will take to deliver the lesson, age of the group, social background, facilities, electric points, any disabilities
   E How many students there will be, the venue, the time it will take to deliver the lesson

5   You have decided to hold a lecture for your next community based project and when explaining this to your manager, they ask for the advantage. From the following options, which option would you tell your manager is an advantage to lectures?

   A Good to use alongside an assessment
   B Very good for one to one interaction
   C Works well combined with an open question assessment
   D Works well for a session with a small child
   E Works well with larger groups

6   You are explaining the process of your sessions to your colleague who has recently taken on the Oral Health Educator role at another practice. Which of the following options explains a lesson evaluation best?

   A Process by which the effects and effectiveness of teaching can be determined
   B Process of determining an outcome
   C Start, middle, end
   D Structure, assessment, outcome
   E Structure, process, outcome

7   You are speaking with your colleague and a dentist at the practice following the most recent oral health educator meeting, The Donabedian concept was discussed in great detail. Which of the following options explains the elements included in the Donabedian concept?

   A Resources, task, outcome
   B Resources, evaluation, outcome
   C Start, middle, assessment, outcome, evaluation
   D Start, middle, end
   E Structure, process, outcome

8   There are many ways you can make assessments on a patient once you have completed a session. An assessment would be completed to understand what has been learned during that session. What types of assessment are correct?

   A Aural, practical, written, and oral
   B Essay, one to one, open questions, observing others
   C Test, demonstration, one to one
   D Written, test, one to one
   E Written essay, practical, and one to one

9 What does OHP stand for?
  A Oral health participants
  B Oral health physics
  C Oral health problems
  D Oral health promises
  E Oral health promotion

10 State the three key domains of learning:
  A Attitude, qualification, and attributes
  B Beliefs, opinions, and behaviour
  C Knowledge, attitude, and behaviour
  D Knowledge, attitude, and skills
  E Skills, knowledge, and behaviour

11 When writing an objective, you must include a verb. From the following options, which answer is a verb?
  A Determine
  B Feel
  C Know
  D State
  E Understand

12 A learner should always reflect on the work they have done. As an oral health educator and dental nurse, you should also self-reflect when completing your personal development plan (PDP). From the following options, what answer explains self-reflection?
  A Identification and exploration of how well, or not so well, the outcome of a certain activity was achieved.
  B Identifying faults in one's own work
  C Identifying and praising oneself when completing a project
  D Reflection of one's own work when carrying out a task
  E Writing down something that you have learnt

13 What does PROM stand for?
  A Patient's realistic objective measures
  B Patient reported objective measures
  C Patient reported outcome measures
  D Primary, realistic, objective, measurement
  E Primary reported objective measurement

14 Your manager has asked for an explanation of what an oral health educator session entails to help a new member of staff. When explaining this to your manager, they ask for the advantage of evaluation through questionnaires. From the following options, what is an advantage of using a questionnaire as an evaluation method?

A Gives immediate feedback and shows results on paper

B Quick response and easy to look at

C Shows results on paper and easy to read

D The patient only answers what they think we want them to answer

E They write down what they believe to be true

Extended Matching Questions

For each of the following questions, select the most appropriate answer from the list below. The answers might be used once, more than once, or not at all.

Topic: Lesson Preparation and Communication

a) Attitude

b) Explanation

c) Interface

d) Positive reinforcement

e) Primary

f) Relevance

g) Secondary

h) Understanding

1 In order for a patient to learn new information, they have to pass through seven steps and changes. Some of these steps are: unawareness, awareness, self-interest, belief, commitment, and action. Which of the options is the most appropriate for the missing step?

2 When giving dental education, you must remember different the points of learning theory. One of the learning theories is described as 'if you tell a patient too many facts all in one go they often get confused'. Which of the options listed would you select as the most appropriate learning theory?

3 You are working alongside a dental nurse who is training to become an oral health educator. You are talking about prevention and the different categories. You provide scenarios and then let the trainee answer which type of prevention it is; the next scenario you give is 'a patient being vaccinated against rubella'. Which of the options listed would you select as the most appropriate type of prevention?

Answers

1   When planning a lesson, you have a lot of things to consider, such as target audience and the topic. From the following options, which are two considerations that need to be taken into account when setting an objective?

Correct Answer: a) Objective needs to be appropriate to the target audience and suitable for the setting

All objectives need to be appropriate to the target group that is being taught. It is no use to state an objective that is completely different to the aim stated. They must be suitable for the setting, e.g. it would be difficult to set an objective of 50 children to all demonstrate toothbrushing techniques at the same time.

2   An objective must be measured to show that the patient has learned. From the following options, how is an objective measured?

Correct Answer: c) By time

An objective is measured by time, hence why the statement most often used is 'By the end of the session the patient will be able to . . .': you are stating a time frame (by the end of the session).

3   A lesson can be planned based on aims and objectives. SMART objectives were created to combine them with the learning outcomes. What does SMART stand for?

Correct Answer: e) Specific, measurable, attainable, relevant, and time related

SMART is used to help create a realistic objective during a lesson.

4   You have been asked to plan a lesson for five patients; before you start creating the lesson plan you have something to consider. Using the following options, what would you consider before starting the lesson plan?

Correct Answer: d) How many students there will be, the venue, the time it will take to deliver the lesson, age of the group, social background, facilities, electrical points, any disabilities

Preparation prior to a lesson is essential to ensure that the lesson goes to plan. It is vital to consider the above. If these are not considered, then the lesson is not planned appropriately, and the desired outcome may be compromised.

5   You have decided to hold a lecture for your next community based project; when explaining this to your manager, they ask for the advantage. From the following options, which option would you tell your manager is an advantage to lectures?

Correct Answer: e) Works well with larger groups

A talk or lecture tends to work better with a larger audience. You are able to get the message across to a large number of people in a direct and monitored way. You would be able to carry out a talk/lecture on a specific subject and then ask the target audience to complete a questionnaire on the topic discussed.

6 You are explaining the process of your sessions to your colleague who has recently taken on the Oral Health Educator role at another practice. Which of the following options explains a lesson evaluation best?

Correct Answer: a) Process by which the effects and effectiveness of teaching can be determined

An evaluation of a lesson is essential to determine if the desired outcome/objective was met. You make a judgement on the effectiveness of the session and state what has worked well/not so well and why this might be.

7 You are speaking with your colleague and a dentist at the practice following the most recent oral health educator meeting, The Donabedian concept was discussed in great detail. Which of the following options explains the elements included in the Donabedian concept?

Correct Answer: e) Structure, process, outcome

The Donabedian concept is a conceptual model that provides a framework for examining health services and evaluating the quality of healthcare. According to the model, information about the quality of care given can be drawn from three categories: 'structure', 'process', and 'outcomes'.

8 There are many ways you can make assessments on a patient once you have completed a session. An assessment would be completed to understand what has been learned during that session. What types of assessment are correct?

Correct Answer: a) Aural, practical, written, and oral

Aural refers to reading. Practical assessments are used to assess skills and behaviours and work best when the task is 'live' and is as close as possible to carrying out the task in an actual circumstance.

9 What does OHP stand for?

Correct Answer: e) Oral health promotion

Oral health promotion involves oral health policies, strategies, and legislative actions where appropriate.

10 State the three key domains of learning:

Correct Answer: c) Knowledge, attitude, and behaviour

The three key domains of learning are based on receiving new information and increasing one's knowledge. After gaining the knowledge then there is a changing of attitudes and/or beliefs. One's behaviour will then be affected as this will improve skills.

11 When writing an objective you must include a verb. From the following options, which answer is a verb?

Correct Answer: d) State

To state something is to formally write or say something. It is a 'doing' word, also known as a verb, and so therefore falls under an objective.

12 A learner should always reflect on the work they have done. As an oral health educator and dental nurse you should also self-reflect when completing your personal development plan (PDP). From the following options, what answer explains self-reflection?

Correct Answer: a) Identification and exploration of how well, or not so well, the outcome of a certain activity was achieved

Self-reflection is an exploration of how well or not so well the outcome of an activity was achieved. This can be done through various processes, e.g. PDP (personal development plan) and reflective writing. It is important to realise when things did not go to plan and reflect on this with an aim to improve it for next time. During oral health education studies and course work, reflective practice plays a big part. You are asked to reflect on your performance and what you feel you did or did not do so well. It is important to reflect and see if there would be any changes made for next time.

13 What does PROM stand for?

Correct Answer: c) Patient reported outcome measures

Patients are asked to complete a pre and post experience questionnaire. This will give the educator feedback and an opportunity to express their opinions. This can be in the form of open or closed questions.

14 Your manager has asked for an explanation of what an oral health educator session entails to help a new member of staff. When explaining this to your manager, they ask for the advantage of evaluation through questionnaires. From the following options, what is an advantage of using a questionnaire as an evaluation method?

Correct Answer: a) Gives immediate feedback and shows results on paper

When using a questionnaire as an evaluation method, it gives immediate feedback and the results will be on paper, which acts as a paper trail. Using this type of evaluation method gives the learner the opportunity to answer questions without the worry of being asked verbally. It is the most popular method of evaluation used and is very often used during exhibitions and displays. The questionnaire will often be given to the learner before they viewed the display/exhibition and then after they have viewed it, to see if they have learnt anything from the display.

Extended Matching Questions

Topic: Lesson preparation and communication

1   In order for a patient to learn new information, they have to pass through seven steps and changes. Some of these steps are: unawareness, awareness, self-interest, belief, commitment, and action. Which of the options is the most appropriate for the missing step?

Correct Answer: a) Attitude

In order for a patient to learn, there are several steps that have to be made with knowledge and behavioural changes.

Unawareness – The patient may be unaware they have a particular problem; therefore, they have no knowledge of how to correct the problem.

Awareness – The patient must be made aware of their problem.

Self-interest – If the problem is made personally relevant to the patient, they will develop self-interest.

Attitude – Once the patient is made aware of the problem and develops self-interest, then their attitude will change to one that will receive new information.

Belief – The patient will believe the new information when they get a positive response, e.g. I brush my gums and now they do not bleed, but when I stop brushing my gums they bleed again.

Commitment – Once the patient starts to put the new information into action, they develop commitment.

Action – Once the patient becomes committed, they then act on the new information.

2   When giving dental education, you must remember different points of learning theory; one of the learning theories is described as 'if you tell a patient too many facts all in one go they often get confused'. Which of the options listed would you select as the most appropriate learning theory?

Correct Answer: c) Interface

When using learning theories, you should follow the points to help patients get the most from the education you are providing.

Information fade – New information is easily and often forgotten; therefore, it is important to keep repeating yourself.

Interference – If you tell a patient too many facts all in one go, they often get confused. Remember one visit = one dental health message.

Positive reinforcement – Tell the patients how well they are doing. This will give them encouragement to carry on.

Interest – If the patients are interested in what they are learning, it gives them motivation to continue learning.

Relevance – The message you are giving to the patient should be relevant. Point out the relevance to the patient, this will help them learn.

Example – It is easier to show the patients how to brush their teeth rather than tell them!

Learning speed – People learn at different rates. Remember that, and adapt the learning pace of the patient for your session to be successful.

Trust – Giving oral health advice can be very personal to the patient. The patient must feel they can trust and not resent you.

3   You are working alongside a dental nurse who is training to become an oral health educator. You are talking about prevention and the different categories. You provide scenarios and then let the trainee answer which type of prevention it is; the next scenario you give is 'a patient being vaccinated against rubella'. Which of the options listed would you select as the most appropriate type of prevention?

Correct Answer: e) Primary

Prevention is separated into three different categories: primary prevention, secondary prevention, and tertiary prevention. Each category is at a different stage in the disease process and each requires different health education input.

Primary prevention – Primary means earliest or first. Information is given on health threats in order to sustain a healthy status and avoid any risks leading to disease.

Secondary prevention – A change of behaviour may be required. People require this prevention when they are at risk from disease or show early symptoms.

Tertiary prevention – This prevention is for the patient who has the disease. The patient needs to recognise the symptoms and take action to cure the disease. A rehabilitation programme needs to be followed to prevent the disease from occurring again.

12

Socio-Economic Classification, Class, and Socialisation

1 What is meant by demography?
   A A study of the age of the population
   B A study by statistical methods of the human population
   C A study by statistical methods of disease
   D A study of dental disease
   E A study of the gender of population

2 The Census is carried out every 10 years by the Office for National Statistics; which of the following does the Census not cover?
   A Educational qualifications
   B Employment
   C Place of residence
   D Place of birth
   E Types of accommodation

3 When referring to the Registrar General's Classifications of Class, which class would a police officer fall under?
   A I
   B II
   C III
   D IV
   E V

4 When referring to the Registrar General's Classifications of Class, which class would a postman fall under?
   A I
   B II
   C III
   D IV
   E V

Questions and Answers in Oral Health Education, First Edition. Chloe Foxhall and Anna Lown.
© 2021 John Wiley & Sons Ltd. Published 2021 by John Wiley & Sons Ltd.
Companion website: www.wiley.com/go/foxhall/oral-health-education

5 When referring to the Registrar General's Classifications of Class, which class would a dentist fall under?

A I

B II

C III

D IV

Extended Matching Questions

For each of the following questions, select the most appropriate answer from the list below. The answers might be used once, more than once, or not at all.

Topic: Socio-economic Classification, Class, and Socialisation

a) Class I
b) Class II
c) Class IV
d) Ethnic background
e) Gender
f) Magazine
g) Parents
h) The Census

1 There are many reasons why patients may be socially disadvantaged. Some of these may be education, parental discipline, and peer group pressure. Which of the options listed is the most appropriate for another reason a patient may be socially disadvantaged?

2 The Registrar General's Classification shows that people who are in the lower classes suffer from higher rates of dental disease. Which of the options listed is the most appropriate for what class these people would be in?

3 There are two types of socialisation: primary socialisation and secondary socialisation. Primary socialisation refers to when a child is learning the basic norms of society. Secondary socialisation refers to a child learning what is acceptable and what is not. From the options listed, which is the most appropriate answer for who could influence the child during secondary socialisation?

Answers

1 What is meant by demography?

Correct Answer: b) A study by statistical methods of the human population

Demography is the study by statistical methods of the human population. Its main concern is the measurement of population changes over a period, the main focus being on births and deaths. Then follows a more detailed description of the population such as sex, age, disease, etc. The main methods of finding out this information are through the census, registration of births, deaths, and marriages, and the Registrar General's Classifications of Class.

2 The Census is carried out every 10 years by the Office for National Statistics, which of the following does the Census not cover?

Correct Answer: d) Place of birth

The Census is very detailed and everyone has to complete it; if they don't they can face fines. The Census remains confidential. The questions asked of the population cover the following subjects: types of accommodation, place of residence, educational qualifications, employment, and transport access.

3 When referring to the Registrar General's Classifications of Class, which class would a police officer fall under?

Correct Answer: c) III – non-manual

The Registrar General's Classifications of Class is broken down into five classes. Class III – non-manual – is related to clerical, skilled manual, and supervisory skills such as clerk, police officer, typist, and draughtsman.

4 When referring to the Registrar General's Classifications of Class, which class would a postman fall under?

Correct Answer: d) IV

The Registrar General's Classifications of Class is broken down into five classes. Class IV is related to semi-skilled or unskilled manual skills such as farm workers, waiting staff, or delivery staff.

5 When referring to the Registrar General's Classifications of Class, which class would a dentist fall under?

Correct Answer: a) I

The Registrar General's Classifications of Class is broken down into five classes. Class I is related to professional skills, such as doctors, dentists, engineers, and directors.

Extended Matching Questions

Topic: Socio-economic Classification, Class, and Socialisation

1   There are many reasons why patients may be socially disadvantaged. Some of these may be education, parental discipline, and peer group pressure. Which of the options listed is the most appropriate for another reason a patient may be socially disadvantaged?

    Correct Answer: d) Ethnic background

    Many factors contribute to patients being at a social disadvantage. Being socially disadvantaged does have an effect on dental disease.

    Wealth – can't afford a toothbrush.

    Education – parents can't read leaflets.

    Single parents – lack of time for self and children.

    Parental discipline – strict parents.

    General health – having sugary medicines and having other worries.

    Peer group pressure – peer pressure to eat the sweets.

    Ethnic background – different eating habits.

    Mental or physical handicap – may not be able to brush teeth.

    Unfluoridated water – especially in the north west of England.

    Size of family – sharing one toothbrush.

    Ignorance – having sweet foods and drinks between meals.

2   The Registrar General's Classification shows that people who are in the lower classes suffer from higher rates of dental disease. Which of the options listed is the most appropriate for what class these people would be in?

    Correct Answer: c) Class IV

    The lower classes such as IV and V are classed as the semi-skilled workers, unskilled manual workers, unskilled workers, or unemployed.

3   There are two types of socialisation: primary socialisation, and secondary socialisation. Primary socialisation refers to when a child is learning the basic norms of society. Secondary socialisation refers to a child learning what is acceptable and what is not. From the options listed, which is the most appropriate answer for who could influence the child during secondary socialisation?

    Correct Answer: f) Magazines

    Secondary socialisation refers to subsequent contacts as the child grows. It mainly occurs when the child attends full-time education. The child learns to be an effective member of society. The child learns what is acceptable and what is not, e.g. how to play games and not be a bully. Health educators must realise peer pressure is very strong and can sometimes overrule what you say.

Others who can influence the child:

- friends
- television
- teachers
- magazine
- radio
- posters
- adverts
- peer groups
- trends
- pop idols.

13

Fluoride and Fissure Sealants

1 Fluoride is known to prevent dental caries, by changing the structure of the enamel, when it is incorporated into the patient's routine. Which of the following is an example of systemic fluoride?
   A Fluoride gel
   B Fluoride mouthwash
   C Fluoride tablets
   D Fluoride toothpaste
   E Fluoride varnish

2 A parent asks the dentist about fluoride drops and how much should be given to the child. The dentist explains that the region they are living in has fluoridated water so this would not be required. Which of the following options shows the amount of fluoride added to in the water supply to in some areas of the UK?
   A 1 ppm
   B 100 ppm
   C 4500 ppm
   D 2800 ppm
   E 10 000 ppm

3 Fluoride application is considered as a method for caries prevention. Which areas of the teeth benefit from these areas?
   A Buccal surfaces
   B Interproximal surfaces
   C Lingual surfaces
   D Occlusal fissures
   E Palatal surfaces

Questions and Answers in Oral Health Education, First Edition. Chloe Foxhall and Anna Lown.
© 2021 John Wiley & Sons Ltd. Published 2021 by John Wiley & Sons Ltd.
Companion website: www.wiley.com/go/foxhall/oral-health-education

4   The enamel of the tooth is made up of crystals; the most common constituents are calcium and phosphate in the form of hydroxyapatite crystals. When fluoride is given systemically or topically, it alters the cell structure of the tooth. An ion exchange takes place. What is the name of the new converted crystals?
   A Fluorapatite crystals
   B Fluorhydroxy crystals
   C Fluoridehydroxy crystals
   D Fluorphosphate crystals
   E Hydroxyfluoride crystals

5   An 11-year-old patient attends the dental practice for an oral health session with her mother. The mum has introduced fluoride mouth rinse as a part of the child's oral hygiene routine to prevent caries. The mum would like to know when the best time is for the child to use the mouth rinse?
   F After brushing
   G At a separate time to brushing
   H Before brushing
   I Instead of brushing
   J Not to be done at all

6   Fluoride, if used incorrectly, can be toxic to a child. If fluoride is swallowed in large doses it can cause serious harm. If this was to happen, the first thing you would do is find how much has been taken and inform the dentist or local hospital. The child who has overdosed is also given something to counteract with fluoride; what would this be?
   A Milk
   B Nothing, this could make the patient sick
   C Oxygen
   D Paracetamol
   E Water

7   The British Fluoridation Society was founded by a group of concerned professionals that wanted to see an improvement in dental health throughout the UK population by the implementation of fluoridated water. What year was the British Fluoridation Society founded?
   A 1960
   B 1969
   C 1973
   D 1980
   E 1984

8   There have been various studies and reports written about fluoride and fluoridation. A report was published on the alleged linkage between human cancer and fluoridation. What was this report called?
   A Department of Health and Social Security Report
   B Fluoridation Review
   C Knox Report
   D McColl Report
   E York Review

9 What statement best describes a fissure sealant?

A composite filling placed over an occlusal surface

B A plastic coating placed on the fissures of the posterior teeth to help prevent caries

C A plastic coating placed on all teeth to help prevent caries

D A plastic filling placed on the fissures of the posterior teeth to help prevent peri-odontal disease

E An amalgam filling placed over an occlusal surface

Extended Matching Questions

For each of the following questions, select the most appropriate answer from the list below. The answers might be used once, more than once, or not at all.

Topic: Fluoride

a) 25%

b) 400–600 ppm

c) 1000 ppm +

d) 1350–1500 ppm

e) Cavity

f) Fluorosis

g) Systemically

h) Topically

1 You have a parent booked in today for an oral health session; the parent has a 2 year old and a 6 year old. You have recommended toothpaste for the 6 year old that contains 1350–1500 ppm fluoride and to use a pea size amount. You recommend that the 2 year old should only use a smear of toothpaste. The water in the area that the family lives in is not fluoridated. Which of the answers is the most appropriate fluoride strength to recommend for the 2 year old?

2 You are discussing an image with a trainee dental nurse from her coursework. A 6-year old-child presents with white spots on the lower first molars that have recently erupted. Which of the answers is the most appropriate explanation for this?

3 A patient has been using fluoride gel as prevention. It was recommended by their dentist as they are a high caries risk patient. Which of the answers is most appropriate for the way this fluoride works?

Answers

1 Fluoride is known to prevent dental caries, by changing the structure of the enamel, when it is incorporated into the patient's routine. Which of the following is an example of systemic fluoride?

Correct Answer: c) Fluoride tablets

Fluoride that is ingested through various products such as tablets, drops, or water and then incorporated into the internal structure of the teeth is classed as systemic. Fluoride that is applied to the surface of the teeth, such as gels or varnishes, is classed as topical.

2 A parent asks the dentist about fluoride drops and how much should be given to the child. The dentist explains that the region they are living in has fluoridated water so this would not be required. Which of the following options shows the amount of fluoride added to in the water supply to in some areas of the UK?

Correct Answer: a) 1 ppm

The amount of fluoride artificially added to the water supply is 1 part per million (PPM). Regions of the country that have this in place have shown incidence of caries in the population to reduce by up to 50%. Higher concentrations could cause overdose and problems such as fluorosis.

3 Fluoride application is considered a method for caries prevention. Which areas on the teeth benefit from these areas?

Correct Answer: b) Interproximal surfaces

All other surfaces listed can be cleaned by a good toothbrushing technique. The interproximal surface can only be cleaned by interproximal cleaning, which is not always completed because these areas present as the more challenging areas to clean. Most white spot lesions or demineralisation lesions begin in these areas first. Applying fluoride to these areas can prevent this.

4 The enamel of the tooth is made up of crystals; the most common constituents are calcium and phosphate in the form of hydroxyapatite crystals. When fluoride is given systemically or topically, it alters the cell structure of the tooth. An ion exchange takes place. What is the name of the new converted crystals?

Correct Answer: a) Fluorapatite crystals

Fluoride alters the cell structure of these crystals from hydroxyapatite to fluorapatite. Fluorapatite is more resistant to acid attacks and therefore works as a caries prevention treatment.

5 An 11-year-old patient attends the dental practice for an oral health session with her mother. The mum has introduced fluoride mouth rinse as part of the child's oral hygiene routine to prevent caries. The mum would like to know when the best time is for the child to mouth rinse.

Correct Answer: b) At a separate time to brushing

A fluoride mouth rinse should be done at a different time to brushing to provide an extra topical coating of fluoride. It should be performed for 1–2 minutes. Fluoride mouth rinse is not recommended for children under the age of 6 years' old. This is to prevent young children swallowing the rinse, which could cause fluorosis.

6 Fluoride, if used incorrectly, can be toxic to a child. If fluoride is swallowed in large doses, it can cause serious harm. If this was to happen, the first thing you would do is find how much has been taken and inform the dentist or local hospital. The child who has overdosed is also given something to counteract with the fluoride; what would this be?

Correct Answer: a) Milk

A child that has overdosed on fluoride should be given milk to drink in copious amounts. This is because calcium absorbs fluoride which will help counteract the effect of the overdose. This could also make the child sick. The patient would then need to attend the hospital for treatment and you, as a dental nurse, would need to write up all relevant records.

7 The British Fluoridation Society was founded by a group of concerned professionals that wanted to see an improvement in dental health throughout the UK population by the implementation of fluoridated water. What year was the British Fluoridation Society founded?

Correct Answer: b) 1969

The British Fluoridation Society was founded in 1969. Founder members include Eric Lubbock MP. The society was keen to include fluoride in the water supply at a safe level to improve dental health in the UK. Fluoride does occur naturally in some water, some cities are naturally fluoridated whereas others are artificially fluoridated.

8 There have been various studies and reports written about fluoride and fluoridation. A report was published on the alleged linkage between human cancer and fluoridation. What was this report called?

Correct Answer: b) Knox Report

The Knox Report was published as a 116-page report on 14 January 1985. The working party was commissioned with the remit of assessing all published evidence on the alleged link between human cancer and fluoridation in 1980. Members of the working party were authorities in epidemiology, cancer research, pathology, statistics, and water treatment.

9 What statement best describes a fissure sealant?

Correct Answer: d) A plastic coating placed on the fissures of the posterior teeth to help prevent caries

Fissure sealants are plastic coatings that are painted onto the fissures of the posterior teeth. The sealant forms a protective layer that keeps food and bacteria from getting stuck in the fissures of the teeth and thus causing caries.

Extended Matching Questions

Topic: Fluoride

1 You have a parent booked in today for an oral health session, the parent has a 2 year old and a 6 year old. You have recommended toothpaste for the 6 year old that contains 1350–1500 ppm fluoride and to use a pea size amount. You recommend that the 2 year old should only use a smear of toothpaste. The water in the area that the family lives in is not fluoridated. Which of the answers is the most appropriate fluoride strength to recommend for the 2 year old?

Correct Answer: c) 1000 ppm +

A child at the age of 2 should be using a smear of toothpaste with at least 1000 ppm fluoride in. A child between the ages of 3 and 6 should be using a pea sized amount of between 1350 and 1500 ppm fluoride toothpaste. A child of this age should always be monitored when using fluoride as if used incorrectly and ingested in large quantities it can be fatal.

2 You are discussing an image with a trainee dental nurse from her coursework. A 6-year-old child presents with white spots on the lower first molars that have recently erupted. Which of the answers is the most appropriate explanation for this?

Correct Answer: f) Fluorosis

White spots that are present on teeth from eruption are most likely going to be fluorosis. Fluorosis is caused by overexposure to fluoride while the teeth are being formed. It appears as white or discoloured patches in the enamel. This cannot be removed by cleaning.

3 A patient has been using fluoride gel as prevention. It was recommended by their dentist as they are a high caries risk patient. Which of the answers is most appropriate for the way this fluoride works?

Correct Answer: h) Topically

Fluoride works either topically or systemically. Topically requires the teeth to be coated with the product, such as a gel or varnish. Systemically requires the person being treated to ingest or swallow the product, such as a tablet. Products like fluoridated milk are applied topically and systemically as they coat the teeth while in the mouth, then once swallowed form a systemic benefit.

14

Oral Conditions and Oral Cancers

1 A 64-year-old male patient attends the dental practice for his regular dental examination. The patient has no complaints. On examination, the dentist diagnoses the patient with a harmless swelling within the tissue of the right mandibular due to an abnormal growth of cells. From the following options, what is the name of the diagnosis?
   A Aphthous ulcers
   B Benign tumour
   C Blocked saliva duct
   D Cyst
   E Malignant tumour

2 A 28-year-old female patient attends the dental practice for her regular dental examination. The patient has no complaints. On examination, the dentist diagnoses the patient with a shallow lesion in the soft tissues. From the following options, what is the name of the diagnosis?
   A Aphthous ulcers
   B Benign tumour
   C Blocked saliva duct
   D Cyst
   E Malignant tumour

3 A 55-year-old male patient attends the dental practice for his dental examination. The patient complains of having a cold sore on his lower lip. The dentist is providing the patient with some advice for the cold sore. From the options below, which is the name of the virus that causes a cold sore?
   A Candida albicans
   B Herpes simplex
   C Herpes varicella
   D Herpes zoster
   E Epstein-barr

Questions and Answers in Oral Health Education, First Edition. Chloe Foxhall and Anna Lown.
© 2021 John Wiley & Sons Ltd. Published 2021 by John Wiley & Sons Ltd.
Companion website: www.wiley.com/go/foxhall/oral-health-education

Extended Matching Questions

For each of the following questions, select the most appropriate answer from the list below. The answers might be used once, more than once, or not at all.

Topic: Oral Conditions and Oral Cancers

a) Aphthous ulcers
b) Angular cheilitis
c) Bruxism
d) Denture stomatitis
e) Herpes simplex virus
f) Oral cancer
g) Thrush
h) Xerostomia

1 A 38-year-old female patient attends the dental practice for a dental examination. The patient complains of white patches on her tongue and some ulcerations on the roof of her mouth. The patient wears a lower denture, replacing her lower molars. Which of the answers is the most appropriate for the patient's oral condition?

2 A 68-year-old male patient attends the dental practice for a dental examination. The patient complains of a sore palate; the patient cannot tell if there is any swelling but cannot wear the full upper acrylic denture comfortably. Which of the answers is the most appropriate for the patient's oral condition?

3 An 82-year-old male patient attends the dental practice for a dental examination. The patient complains of sore corners of the mouth; they appear red and cracked. Which of the answers is the most appropriate for the patient's oral condition?

4 A 28-year-old female patient attends the dental practice for a dental examination. The patient complains of a sore lump in her mouth; it appears to be white with a red area surrounding it. Which of the answers is the most appropriate for the patient's oral condition?

5 A 50-year-old male patient attends the dental practice for a dental examination. The patient complains of a cluster of grey ulcers on the lower lip; it started off as a tingling sensation. Which of the answers is the most appropriate for the patient's oral condition?

6 A patient attends the dental practice for the first time, he completed his medical and social history. The dentist reviews these before calling the patient into the surgery. The patient drinks 35–50 units of alcohol a week and smokes 20 cigarettes a day. The dentist decides cessation advice for alcohol and tobacco use. Which of the answers is the most appropriate for the condition the dentist is trying to avoid for this patient?

Answers

1 A 64-year-old male patient attends the dental practice for his regular dental examination. The patient has no complaints. On examination, the dentist diagnoses the patient with a harmless swelling within the tissue of the right mandibular due to an abnormal growth of cells. From the following options, which is the name of the diagnosis?

Correct Answer: b) Benign tumour

A benign tumour is an abnormal growth of cells which is harmless and lacks ability to spread to neighbouring tissue throughout the body; whereas a malignant tumour does cause harm to the body and has the ability to spread to neighbouring tissue throughout the body. A cyst is an abnormal sack of fluid that is located in the tissue. A blocked salivary duct can present as a small lump in the cheek or sublingually. This is usually harmless and will usually disappear by itself. Aphthous ulcers are presented as small shallow lesions that develop on the soft tissues.

2 A 28-year-old female patient attends the dental practice for her regular dental examination. The patient has no complaints. On examination, the dentist diagnoses the patient with a shallow lesion in the soft tissues. From the following options, which is the name of the diagnosis?

Correct Answer: a) Aphthous ulcers

Aphthous ulcers are presented as small shallow lesions that develop on the soft tissues. It is a raw break in the skin and can be quite painful. A benign tumour is an abnormal growth of cells which is harmless and lacks ability to spread to neighbouring tissue throughout the body; whereas a malignant tumour does cause harm to the body and has the ability to spread to neighbouring tissue throughout the body. A cyst is an abnormal sack of fluid that is located in the tissue. A blocked salivary duct can present as a small lump in the cheek or sublingually, it is usually harmless and will usually disappear by itself.

3 A 55-year-old male patient attends the dental practice for his dental examination. The patient complains of having a cold sore on his lower lip. The dentist is providing the patient with some advice for the cold sore. From the options below, which option is the name of the virus that causes a cold sore?

Correct Answer: b) Herpes simplex

Herpes simplex is a virus that remains dormant in the nerve tissue and appears as a cold sore, usually when the person infected suffers stress or the immune system is lowered. Herpes zoster and varicella are the viruses that causes chickenpox and shingles. Epstein-barr is the virus that causes glandular fever. *Candida albicans* is a fungal infection that causes oral thrush.

Extended Matching Questions

For each of the following questions, select the most appropriate answer from the list below. The answers might be used once, more than once or not at all.

Topic: Oral Conditions and Oral Cancers

1 A 38-year-old female patient attends the dental practice for a dental examination. The patient complains of white patches on her tongue and some ulcerations on the roof of her mouth. The patient wears a lower denture replacing her lower molars. Which of the answers is the most appropriate for the patient's oral condition?

Correct Answer: g) Thrush

Oral thrush is a fungal infection that is characterised by white patches and ulcerations of the tongue or other oral mucosal surfaces which can be wiped off with gauze. It is caused by infection with the microorganism *candida albicans*. It is treated with anti-fungal treatments such as mouthwash or lozenges. If thrush is left untreated it can cause angular cheilitis.

2 A 68-year-old male patient attends the dental practice for a dental examination. The patient complains of a sore palate; the patient cannot tell if there is any swelling but cannot wear the full upper acrylic denture comfortably. Which of the answers is the most appropriate for the patient's oral condition?

Correct Answer: d) Denture stomatitis

Denture stomatitis is inflammation of the mouth. This is commonly caused by poor cleaning of the dentures and can lead to infections and inflammations. A denture being left in overnight can also cause thrush infections. It may start as a red patch on the palate and is commonly described as being uncomfortable. If it is left untreated, then it can become painful. Patients must remove their dentures at night and clean them thoroughly. The infection would be treated the same way that thrush is treated. Stomatitis can also have some cases related to poor diet, anaemia, diabetes, or HIV/AIDS.

3 An 82-year-old male patient attends the dental practice for a dental examination. The patient complains of sore corners of the mouth; they appear red and cracked. Which of the answers is the most appropriate for the patient's oral condition?

Correct Answer: f) Angular cheilitis

Angular cheilitis presents itself as red, cracking of radiating fissures from the corners of the mouth. It is sometimes covered with a white membrane which can be wiped off. It normally accompanies intra-oral candidiasis. It is treated with an antifungal cream on the external surfaces, on the internal surfaces it should be treated with a mouthwash or lozenge. It is more common in elderly patients.

4 A 28-year-old female patient attends the dental practice for a dental examination. The patient complains of a sore lump in her mouth; it appears to be white with a red area surrounding it. Which of the answers is the most appropriate for the patient's oral condition?

Correct Answer: a) Aphthous ulcers

Aphthous ulcers can occur singularly or in clusters on the lips or the cheeks of the oral mucosa. They take around 10 days to heal. Most cases are related to anaemia, diabetes, stress, or other medical conditions. A major aphthous ulcer is one singular large ulcer that can take up to a month to heal and can leave a scar.

5 A 50-year-old male patient attends the dental practice for a dental examination. The patient complains of a cluster of grey ulcers on the lower lip; it started off as a tingling sensation. Which of the answers is the most appropriate for the patient's oral condition?

Correct Answer: e) Herpes simplex virus

Herpes simplex type 1, also known as a cold sore, is likely to start during childhood. The virus infects through moist inner skin that lines the mouth. It is commonly passed on by skin contact, such as kissing. It is a viral infection that starts as a tingling or burning sensation that then develops grey ulcers in a cluster. The virus can lie dormant for years and cause no symptoms and then becomes active; cold sores can be triggered by sunshine, stress, illness, and menstruation.

6 A patient attends the dental practice for the first time; he completed his medical and social history. The dentist reviews these before calling the patient into the surgery. The patient drinks 35–50 units of alcohol a week and smokes 20 cigarettes a day. The dentist decides cessation advice for alcohol and tobacco use. Which of the answers is the most appropriate for the condition the dentist is trying to avoid for this patient?

Correct Answer: f) Oral cancer

Oral cancer has lots of risk factors, two of the biggest which are usually related are alcohol and tobacco use. Alcohol is thought to promote carcinogenesis by a number of mechanisms for example; alcohol penetrates the effects of topical carcinogens, such as those found in tobacco. Quitting smoking causes a sharp decrease in oral and pharyngeal cancer. Other risk factors are sunlight, nutrition, infective causes, and oncogenes.

15

Legislation and GDC Standards

1 As a GDC registrant, you are expected to abide by various publications while working in dentistry. Which of the following is not one of these publications?
 A BDA Good Practice
 B GDC publication Preparing for Practice
 C GDC publication Scope of Practice
 D HTM 01-05
 E Standards of the Dental Team

2 You are nursing for a dentist who has submitted false basic periodontal examinations (BPEs) for multiple patients. You have reported this to your Senior Dentist and Practice Manager; which of the following legislations would protect you during the process?
 A General Data Protection Regulations 2018
 B Health and Safety Act 1974
 C Mental Capacity Act 2005
 D Public Interest Disclosure Act 1998
 E Safeguarding Vulnerable Adults Group 2006

3 A 14-year-old male attends the dental practice for a pain appointment; the patient showed a good degree of understanding and knowledge. He attended with his grandmother. What legislation would you refer to?
 A Duty of Candour
 B Freedom of Information Act 2000
 C Gillick Competence
 D Mental Capacity Act 2005
 E The Care Act 2014

Questions and Answers in Oral Health Education, First Edition. Chloe Foxhall and Anna Lown.
© 2021 John Wiley & Sons Ltd. Published 2021 by John Wiley & Sons Ltd.
Companion website: www.wiley.com/go/foxhall/oral-health-education

4 As an oral health educator, you will be expected to visit community places such as schools and care homes; it is extremely important to keep up to date details of record keeping, confidentiality, and data security and protection. Which GDC Standard would you refer to for record keeping, confidentiality, and data security and protection?

A Principle 1
B Principle 3
C Principle 4
D Principle 5
E Principle 8

5 As an oral health educator, you will be expected to visit community places such as schools and care homes. It is extremely important to know how to raise concerns if you come across any. The way of doing so may be different to when you are in practice, but is equally important and should not be ignored as this is part of your professional duty. Which GDC Standard would you refer to for raising concerns if patients are at risk?

A Principle 2
B Principle 4
C Principle 6
D Principle 8
E Principle 9

6 When dealing with usage and storage of data, it is extremely important to follow regulations that are published to guide you as a professional. Which regulation would you refer to for information on collecting, use, storage, and disposal of personal information?

A Access to Health Records 1990
B Data Protection Act 1998
C Freedom of Information Act 2000
D GDPR 2018
E Health and Social Care Act 2008

Extended Matching Questions

For each of the following questions, select the most appropriate answer from the list below. The answers might be used once, more than once, or not at all.

Topic: Legislation

a) Amendment Order 2005
b) Caldicott Regulations
c) Data Protection Act 1998
d) General Data Protection Regulations 2018
e) General Dental Council
f) Mental Capacity Act 2005
g) Public Interest Disclosure Act 1998
h) Scope of Practice

1 Legislation is in place to ensure the security of patient's personal information. It also stops dental practices sending the information to a third party without consent from the patient. From the options listed, which is the most appropriate and up-to-date legislation that prevents these things from happening?

2 You are speaking to a dental nurse on your lunch break and she reveals concerns about the dentist she is working with; she states that the dentist is claiming for treatment that he is not completing on multiple patients. You instruct the dental nurse to report this immediately. Which of the options listed is the most appropriate legislation to protect you from any retaliation during this incident report?

Answers

1 As a GDC registrant, you are expected to abide by various publications while working in dentistry; which of the following is not one of these publications?

Correct Answer: a) BDA Good Practice

The BDA Good Practice document was published by the BDA for gold standard practice, not essential practice. The GDC Standards, Preparing for Practice and Scope of Practice are published to set a standard that all registrants have to abide by to gain and keep registration.

2 You are nursing for a dentist who has submitted false basic periodontal examinations (BPEs) for multiple patients, you have reported this to your Senior Dentist and Practice Manager. Which of the following legislations would protect you during the process?

Correct Answer: d) Public Interest Disclosure Act 1998

The Public Interest Disclosure Act protects employees that raise concerns or whistle blow on an employer or prescribed person within the workplace. When reporting a colleague in the interest of the patients, it may also be referred to as whistle blowing.

3 A 14-year-old male attends the dental practice for a pain appointment; the patient showed a good degree of understanding and knowledge. He attended with his grandmother. What legislation would you refer to?

Correct Answer: c) Gillick Competence

In this situation, as the patient is under 16, you have the ability to assess the patient's Gillick Competence. If they are showing full understanding of the treatment being proposed to them and all the risks and benefits included, then an under 16 year old can consent to dental treatment. This is accepted by the law and cannot be overruled by a parent or guardian.

4 As an oral health educator, you will be expected to visit community places such as schools and care homes, it is extremely important to keep up to date details of record keeping, confidentiality, and data security and protection. Which GDC Standard would you refer to for record keeping, confidentiality, and data security and protection?

Correct Answer: c) Principle 4

Principle 4 states the patient expects their records to be up to date, complete, clear, accurate, and legible, that their personal details are kept confidential, to be able to access their dental records, and their records to be stored securely.

5 As an oral health educator, you will be expected to visit community places such as schools and care homes. It is extremely important to know how to raise concerns if you come across any. The way of doing so may be different to when you are in practice, but is equally important and should not be ignored as this is part of your professional duty. Which GDC Standard would you refer to for raising concerns if patients are at risk?

Correct Answer: d) Principle 8

Principle 8 states the patient expects the dental team to act promptly to protect their safety if there are any concerns raised. It is expected that concerns would be raised about the welfare of vulnerable patients.

6 When dealing with usage and storage of data, it is extremely important to follow regulations that are published to guide you as a professional. Which regulation would you refer to for information on collecting, use, storage, and disposal of personal information?

Correct Answer: d) GDPR 2018

The General Data Protection Regulations were introduced in 2018 for organisations to be more accountable for personal information and the way it is handled. It also gives individuals more control over how their information is used and/or shared. Its main purpose is to control unauthorised sharing of personal information for marketing purposes.

Extended Matching Questions

Topic: Legislation and GDC Standards

1 Legislation is in place to ensure the security of patient's personal information. It also stops dental practices sending the information to a third party without consent from the patient. From the options listed, which is the most appropriate and up-to-date legislation that prevents these things from happening?

Correct Answer: d) General Data Protection Regulations 2018

General Data Protection Regulations were put in place in 2018 to replace the Data Protection Act 1998. GDPR aims to protect all confidentiality of personal data of patients and employees. GDPR gives a person more control over how their information is handled.

2 You are speaking to a dental nurse on your lunch break and she reveals concerns about the dentist she is working with; she states that the dentist is claiming for treatment that he is not completing on multiple patients. You instruct the dental nurse to report this immediately. Which of the options listed is the most appropriate legislation to protect you from any retaliation during this incident report?

Correct Answer: g) Public Interest Disclosure Act 1998

Under these circumstances, an employee that raises a genuine concern about any issue that can affect the public would be protected from any retaliation by the Public Interest Disclosure Act.

16

Screening, Surveys, Indices, Epidemiology, Prevalence, and Incidence

1 What best describes incidence?
   A The cause behind disease
   B The cause of something, e.g. the cause of caries is sugar
   C The incidence and distribution of disease
   D The occurrence of something, e.g. caries, periodontal disease, etc.
   E The process of examining a large proportion of the population

2 What best describes epidemiology?
   A Surveying the area for research purposes
   B The cause behind disease
   C The study of incidence and distribution of disease in large populations
   D The study of occurrence
   E The process of examining a small proportion of the population

3 What best describes aetiology?
   A The occurrence of dental caries
   B The occurrence of periodontal disease
   C The regulation of the DMF system
   D The science that deals with the causes or origin of disease
   E The study of occurrence

4 What best describes screening?
   A The occurrence of aetiology
   B The occurrence of disease
   C The screening of the whole population
   D The study of disease
   E This is the process of examining a large proportion of the population to determine an outcome

Questions and Answers in Oral Health Education, First Edition. Chloe Foxhall and Anna Lown.
© 2021 John Wiley & Sons Ltd. Published 2021 by John Wiley & Sons Ltd.
Companion website: www.wiley.com/go/foxhall/oral-health-education

5 What best describes prevalence?
  A The study of caries
  B The study of disease
  C The study of occurrence
  D The science that deals with the causes of origin of disease
  E This relates to the existence of something, e.g. where the disease is

6 What best describes a survey?
  A A general look at something or to scan the condition of something
  B A look in depth at a certain condition
  C To record details of dental professionals
  D To survey disease
  E To take surveys of patients

7 What best describes incidence?
  A Relates to any guidance produced on how to measure the occurrence of something
  B Relates to any guidance produced on how to measure the quantity of something
  C Relates to guidance produced about the surveys of dental disease
  D Relates to the existence of something, e.g. where the disease is
  E Relates to the study of occurrence within the dental sector

Extended Matching Question

For each of the following questions, select the most appropriate answer from the list below. The answers might be used once, more than once, or not at all.

Topic: Screening, Surveys, Indices, Epidemiology, Prevalence, and Incidence

a) Aetiology
b) Basic Periodontal Examination
c) Diagnosis
d) DMFT
e) Epidemiology
f) Silnes and Löe plaque Index

1 Governments and local authorities plan preventative measures for future generations. In order to do this they must have details of the presence of a disease along with information on the severity, spread and origins of the disease. What is the name given to the type study that will provide this information?

2 Dentists are advised to routinely record data that allows them to highlight areas of particular periodontal activity that the patient needs to address. This data can be used during planning of oral health education sessions to develop outcomes for individual patients. From the list above select the most appropriate form of index that would be useful to the oral health educator.

Answers

1 What best describes incidence?

Correct Answer: d) The occurrence of something, e.g. caries, periodontal disease, etc.

The incidence (occurrence) with regard to dentistry relates to the number of people showing signs of dental disease, e.g. caries, periodontal disease, etc.

2 What best describes epidemiology?

Correct Answer: c) The study of incidence and distribution of disease in large populations

This involves the study of incidence and distribution of disease in large populations, and the conditions influencing the spread and severity of disease.

An example of epidemiology is the 5-year-old dental examination in schools – this is carried out nationally. The teeth are examined for how many are decayed, missing, or filled (DMF).

3 What best describes aetiology?

Correct Answer: d) The science that deals with the causes or origin of disease

This word is mainly used in medicine, where it is the science that deals with the causes or origin of disease; the factors which produce or predispose towards a certain disease or disorder. Simply put, it means the cause behind the disease, e.g. sugar consumption in caries and plaque retention in periodontal disease.

4 What best describes screening?

Correct Answer: e) This is the process of examining a large proportion of the population to determine an outcome

This is the process of examining a large proportion of the population to determine an outcome, e.g. school dental inspection screening.

5 What best describes prevalence?

Correct Answer: e) This relates to the existence of something, e.g. where the disease is

This relates to the existence of caries, periodontal disease, etc. (where it is).

6 What best describes a survey?

Correct Answer: a) A general look at something or to scan the condition of something

A survey is to take a general look at something or to scan the condition of something. A survey is normally carried out for a specific reason, e.g. the study of dental services available for the housebound or for a particular audit.

7 What best describes incidence?

Correct Answer: b) Relates to any guidance produced on how to measure the quantity of something

This simply relates to any guidance produced on how to measure the quantity of something, e.g. the quantity of plaque measured by scoring.

Extended Matching Questions

1 Governments and local authorities plan preventative measures for future generations. In order to do this they must have details of the presence of a disease along with information on the severity, spread and origins of the disease. What is the name given to the type study that will provide this information?

Correct Answer: e) Epidemiology

Epidemiology is the study of distribution and causes of health related events in populations. The Government and local authorities will use this data for analysis and statistical data gathering.

2 Dentists are advised to routinely record data that allows them to highlight areas of particular periodontal activity that the patient needs to address. This data can be used during planning of oral health education sessions to develop outcomes for individual patients. From the list above select the most appropriate form of index that would be useful to the oral health educator.

Correct answer: b) Basic Periodontal Examination

A Basic Periodontal Examination is a form of dental charting that is a screening tool to indicate any area requiring further investigation, advice and treatment.

17

General Health

1 Promoting public health programmes that are put in place is important; to be able to do this, you need to understand them and what they are put in place for. What is the '5 a day' programme the government has put in place?

   A A programme that promotes five appointments at the dentist and ensure good oral health

   B A programme that promotes five hours of dentistry a day to allow DCPs the knowledge required to work in the industry.

   C A programme that promotes five minutes of eating fruit or vegetables to gain a healthy body

   D A programme that promotes five minutes of exercise a day to create good health benefits

   E A programme that promotes five pieces of fruit or vegetable per day thus creating health benefits

2 The body requires essential nutrients to function correctly. Which of the following is not an essential nutrient?

   A Carbohydrates

   B Fibre

   C Fat

   D Mineral

   E Protein

3 Minerals are essential to help the body function. Which of the following is a mineral?

   A Folic acid

   B Niacin

   C Potassium

   D Riboflavin

   E Sorbitol

Questions and Answers in Oral Health Education, First Edition. Chloe Foxhall and Anna Lown.
© 2021 John Wiley & Sons Ltd. Published 2021 by John Wiley & Sons Ltd.
Companion website: www.wiley.com/go/foxhall/oral-health-education

4 Minerals have many benefits for the body. Which of the following is a reason that minerals are essential for the body?

A To burn more calories to aid weight loss
B To help blood pump around the body
C To help with digestion of food
D To maintain the bodies temperature
E To turn the food we eat into energy

5 The body has two different categories of fats. Which of the following is a fat type?

A Fluor-saturates
B Hypo-saturates
C Hypo-unsaturates
D Monofluor-saturates
E Saturates

6 Unsaturated fats are broken down into two types. Which of the following options are the two types of unsaturates?

A Hypo-saturates and hypo-unsaturates
B Hypo-saturates and mono-fluorsaturates
C Hypo-unsaturates and fluor-saturates
D Monofluor-saturates and fluor-saturates
E Polyunsaturates and monounsaturates

7 Saturated fat and unsaturated fat are found in different places. Which of the following options is a place you would find saturates?

A Confectionary
B Fish
C Fruit
D Nuts
E Meat

8 There are two categories of vitamins. Which of the following options are the two types of vitamins?

A Fat-soluble and mono-soluble
B Fat-soluble and water-soluble
C Fluoride-soluble and mono-soluble
D Fluoride-soluble and water-soluble
E Water-soluble and hypo-soluble

9 Fat-soluble vitamins are found in fatty foods such as animal fats and oils; your body needs these vitamins in small amounts to work properly. Which of the following options is a fat-soluble vitamin?

A Biotin
B Magnesium
C Sulphate
D Vitamin D
E Vitamin F

10 Water-soluble vitamins are not stored in the body so you need to have them more frequently. If you have more than you need, your body gets rid of the extra vitamins when you urinate. Which of the following options is a water-soluble vitamin?

A Polyunsaturate

B Vitamin B13

C Vitamin C

D Vitamin D

E Vitamin E

11 Carbohydrates are found in foods like pasta, potato, and bread. From the following options, what are carbohydrates used for within the body?

A To break down sugars

B To help bones grow stronger

C To give the body energy

D To keep us fuller for longer

E To make the body more resistance to microbial attack

12 Protein is essential for the growth and repair of the body. Which of the following options is the percentage of our diet that should be protein?

A 15%

B 25%

C 30%

D 40%

E 50%

13 Dental disease can be connected to bad nutrition. From the following options, which two dental diseases are linked to bad nutrition?

A Cancer and smoker's keratosis

B Caries and smoker's keratosis

C Periodontal disease and caries

D Periodontal disease and halitosis

E Necrotising ulcerative gingivitis and caries

14 What does DEFRA stand for?

A Department for Environment, Food, and Rural Affairs

B Department of Education, Food, and Rural Affairs

C Department of Environmental Fisheries and Rural Affairs

D Department of Environment, Food, Fisheries, and Rural Affairs

E Department of Food and Rural Affairs

15 What does MAFF stand for?

A Ministry of Agriculture, Famine, and Farming

B Ministry of Agriculture, Fisheries, and Food

C Ministry of Appropriate Fisheries and Farming

D Minister of Artificial Food Factories

E Ministry of Famine and Food

16 What does SACN stand for?

  A Science of Advice in Children's Nutrition

  B Scientific Advice Committee on Nutritional Aspects

  C Scientific Advice on the Communication of Nutritional Aspects

  D Scientific Advisory Committee on Nutrition

  E Scientific Advisory of the Communication of Nutrition

17 The government has an eight-point guideline on how to enjoy a healthy diet. Which of the following options are two of the eight in the government's guide for a healthy diet?

  A Don't have sugary foods too often; and eat two lots of fruit per day

  B Eat fruit and vegetables at least twice a day; and enjoy alcohol sensibly

  C Eat raw vegetables; and enjoy alcohol daily

  D Enjoy food; and eat a good portion of carbohydrates

  E If you drink alcohol, drink responsibly and eat a variety of different foods

18 What does NICE stand for?

  A National Indices for Clinical Excellence

  B National Interpretation of Clinical Excellence

  C National Institute for Clinical Excellence

  D National Institute for Health and Clinical Excellence

  E National Institution for Clinical Excellence

19 What is primary care?

  A Care generally described as front-line service, which includes GPs and dentists

  B Care generally described as the first treatment you receive

  C The first care you receive

  D The first and only treatment and care received

  E The care you receive as you enter the care sector, e.g. reception

20 What is secondary care?

  A Care given in the private sector

  B Emergency or specialist care

  C The second visit to the dental practitioner

  D The second visit for treatment to be carried out

  E The second stage of endodontic treatment

Extended Matching Questions

For each of the following questions, select the most appropriate answer from the list below. The answers might be used once, more than once, or not at all.

Topic: General Health

a) Carbohydrates
b) Phosphorous
c) Proteins
d) Riboflavin
e) Vitamin A
f) Vitamin D
g) Vitamin E
h) Vitamin K

1 The body contains fat-soluble vitamins and water-soluble vitamins which provide different benefits to the body. Water-soluble vitamins are not stored in the body and are therefore required more frequently. From the options listed, which is a water-soluble vitamin?

2 Minerals are necessary for three main reasons: turning the food we eat into energy, controlling body fluids inside and outside the body, and building strong bones and teeth. From the options listed, which is a mineral?

Answers

1 Promoting public health programmes that are put in place is important. To be able to do this, you need to understand them and what they are put in place for. What is the '5 a day' programme the government has put in place?

Correct Answer: e) A programme that promotes five pieces of fruit or vegetable a day to create health benefits

The government started a programme which aims to increase fruit and vegetable consumption, thus leading to a healthier lifestyle and helping to prevent disease/illness.

2 The body requires essential nutrients to function correctly. Which of the following is not an essential nutrient?

Correct Answer: b) Fibre

Fibre is not an essential nutrient. The essential nutrients are:

minerals
fats
vitamins
carbohydrates
proteins.

3 Minerals are essential to help the body function. Which of the following is a mineral?

Correct Answer: c) Potassium

Potassium is a mineral that the body uses as an electrolyte, which helps regulate bodily fluid, nerve signals, and muscle contractions.

4 Minerals have many benefits for the body. Which of the following is a reason that minerals are essential for the body?

Correct Answer: e) Turn the food we eat into energy

Minerals are essential to the body for three reasons, one being that they help turn the food we eat into energy. The others are that they help control body fluids inside and outside cells and help with building strong bones and teeth.

5 The body has two different categories of fats. Which of the following is a fat type?

Correct Answer: e) Saturates

Saturates are the type of fats that are bad for us. Saturated fats also contain cholesterol, which clogs up the arteries leading to the heart. The other type of fat is unsaturated, which can be found in oils, fish, and corn.

6 Unsaturated fats are broken down into two types. Which of the following options are the two types of unsaturates?

Correct Answer: e) Polyunsaturates and monounsaturates

Polyunsaturated fat can be found in plant and animal foods, such as salmon, vegetable oils, and some nuts and seeds. Monounsaturates can be found in plant foods, nuts, avocados, and vegetable oil.

7 Saturated fat and unsaturated fat are found in different places. Which of the following options is a place you would find saturates?

Correct Answer: a) Confectionary

Saturated fat is often found in confectionery, such as cakes, chocolates, sweets, and sweet pastries. These are what we should eat less of to maintain a balanced diet.

8 There are two categories of vitamins. Which of the following options are the two types of vitamins?

Correct Answer: b) Fat-soluble and water-soluble

Water soluble vitamins are those that dissolve in water and readily absorb into tissues for immediate use. Because they are not stored in the body, they need to be replenished regularly in our diet. Any excess of water soluble vitamins is quickly excreted in urine and will rarely accumulate to toxic levels. The fat soluble vitamins – A, D, E, and K – are stored in the body for long periods of time and generally pose a greater risk for toxicity when consumed in excess than water soluble vitamins.

9 Fat-soluble vitamins are found in fatty foods such as animal fats and oils; your body needs these vitamins in small amounts to work properly. Which of the following options is a fat soluble vitamin?

Correct Answer: d) Vitamin D

Vitamin D helps regulate the amount of calcium and phosphate in the body. These nutrients are needed to keep bones, teeth, and muscles healthy. A lack of vitamin D can lead to bone deformities, such as rickets in children, and bone pain caused by a condition called osteomalacia in adults.

10 Water-soluble vitamins are not stored in the body, so you need to have them more frequently. If you have more than you need, your body gets rid of the extra vitamins when you urinate. Which of the following options is a water soluble vitamin?

Correct Answer: c) Vitamin C

Water soluble vitamins dissolve in water and are not stored by the body. Since they are eliminated in urine, we require a continuous daily supply in our diet. The water soluble vitamins include the vitamin B-complex group and vitamin C.

11 Carbohydrates are found in foods like pasta, potato, and bread. From the following options, what are carbohydrates used for within the body?

Correct Answer: c) To give the body energy

Although carbohydrates are needed for the body's energy, they are not considered absolutely essential because protein can be converted for this purpose.

12 Protein is essential for the growth and repair of the body. Which of the following options is the percentage of our diet that should be protein?

Correct Answer: a) 15%

Protein is essential for growth and repair of the body; 15% of the calories we eat daily should be from proteins. Proteins include:

- soya
- eggs
- pulses (beans and lentils)
- seeds and nuts
- mycoprotein (Quorn)
- wheat proteins, e.g. bread, rice, and maize
- milk
- dairy products.

13 Dental disease can be connected to bad nutrition. From the following options, which two dental diseases are linked to bad nutrition?

Correct Answer: c) Periodontal disease and caries

Dental diseases include dental caries, developmental defects of enamel, dental erosion, and periodontal disease. The main cause of tooth loss is dental caries in which diet plays an important role. Both periodontal disease and caries are affected by bad nutrition.

14 What does DEFRA stand for?

Correct Answer: a) Department for Environment, Food, and Rural Affairs

This is the UK government department responsible for safeguarding our natural environment, supporting our world-leading food and farming industry, and sustaining a thriving rural economy. Its broad remit means it plays a major role in people's day-to-day life, from the food we eat, and the air we breathe, to the water we drink.

15 What does MAFF stand for?

Correct Answer: b) Ministry of Agriculture, Fisheries, and Food

Responsibilities include:

- better regulation;
- fisheries;
- food and farming, including CAP (Common Agricultural Policy), apprenticeships, exports, and bovine TB (tuberculosis) policy;
- science and innovation.

16 What does SACN stand for?

Correct Answer: d) Scientific Advisory Committee on Nutrition

SACN advises on nutrition and related health matters. It advises Public Health England and other UK government organisations.

17 The government has an eight-point guideline on how to enjoy a healthy diet. Which of the following options are two of the eight in the government's guide to a healthy diet?

Correct Answer: e) If you drink alcohol, drink responsibly; and eat a variety of different foods

- To keep health risks from drinking alcohol to a low level you are safest not regularly drinking more than 14 units per week – 14 units is equivalent to a bottle and a half of wine or five pints of export-type lager (5% abv) over the course of a week – this applies to both men and women.
- If you do drink as much as 14 units per week, it is best to spread this evenly over three days or more.
- If you have one or two heavy drinking sessions, you increase your risks of death from long-term illnesses and from accidents and injuries.
- The risk of developing a range of illnesses (including, for example, cancers of the mouth, throat, and breast) increases with any amount you drink on a regular basis.
- If you wish to cut down the amount you're drinking, a good way to achieve this is to have several alcohol-free days each week.

Eating a variety of different foods: to have a healthy, balanced diet, people should try to eat at least five portions of a variety of fruit and vegetables a day, base meals on starchy foods like potatoes, bread, rice, or pasta, eat some beans, pulses, fish, eggs, meat, and other protein.

18 What does NICE stand for?

Correct Answer: d) National Institute for Health and Clinical Excellence

The National Institute for Health and Care Excellence (NICE) is a non-departmental public body of the Department of Health in the United Kingdom which publishes guidelines in four areas:

- The use of health technologies within the National Health Service (NHS) which looks at the use of new and existing medicines, treatments and procedures.
- Clinical practice.
- Guidance for public sector workers.
- Guidance for social care services and users.

19 What is primary care?

Correct Answer: a) Care generally described as front-line service which includes GPs and dentists

Primary care is generally regarded as a front-line service. It is the first point of contact for most people and is delivered by a wide range of independent contractors such as GPs, dentists, opticians, and pharmacists.

20   What is secondary care?

Correct Answer: b) Emergency or specialist care

Secondary care is known better as acute health care and can be either elective care or emergency care. Elective care means planned specialist medical care from a primary or community health professional, such as a GP.

Extended Matching Questions

Topic: General Health

1   The body contains fat-soluble vitamins and water-soluble vitamins which provide different benefits to the body. Water-soluble vitamins are not stored in the body and are therefore required more frequently. From the options listed, which is a water-soluble vitamin?

Correct Answer: d) Riboflavin

Riboflavin is a water-soluble vitamin along with vitamin B6, vitamin C, vitamin B12, folic acid, biotin, niacin, pantothenic acid, and thiamine. These should be taken into our body regularly as they dissolve in water instantly and are absorbed into tissues for immediate use.

2   Minerals are necessary for three main reasons: turning the food we eat into energy, controlling body fluids inside and outside the body, and building strong bones and teeth. From the options listed, which is a mineral?

Correct Answer: b) Phosphorous

Minerals are important in a well-functioning body. The other essential minerals are: iron, magnesium, calcium, potassium, sodium, and sulphur. Minerals help our body grow, develop, and stay healthy.

18

Medical Emergencies

1 A patient comes into surgery and says they have a pain in their chest; you check the medical history and it is clear, the patient appears pale but responding well. What do you do?
  A Give them oxygen and sit them in the waiting room until their appointment
  B Make the patient comfortable, ask for help and prepare for Basic Life Support.
  C Nothing, they don't have any known medical conditions
  D Offer to lay them down in the chair, it may be they came in from the cold and the heat inside has made them feel unwell
  E Tell the patient to rebook their appointment and to go home and rest

2 A patient attends the dental practice and hands you an updated medical history; you notice the patient is taking metformin, what condition is this medication used for?
  A Epilepsy
  B High blood pressure
  C High cholesterol
  D Low blood pressure
  E Type 2 diabetes

3 You are training a member of staff on medical emergencies; when talking about cardiac arrest, you explain the CPR ratio. What is the CPR ratio on an adult?
  A 10 : 1
  B 15 : 2
  C 20 : 2
  D 30 : 2
  E 30 : 6

4 A patient who is known for having epilepsy has a seizure while waiting for his exam appointment. Which of the following is not a sign for a seizure?
  A Convulsive moments
  B Feeling hungry
  C Incontinence
  D Loss of consciousness
  E Rigidity

Questions and Answers in Oral Health Education, First Edition. Chloe Foxhall and Anna Lown.
© 2021 John Wiley & Sons Ltd. Published 2021 by John Wiley & Sons Ltd.
Companion website: www.wiley.com/go/foxhall/oral-health-education

5 During paediatric CPR, how many breaths are given before compressions are started?

A 1

B 2

C 3

D 4

E 5

6 A patient had a simple extraction of the lower left second molar; it was the last appointment of the day and the patient had come straight from work. As the patient begins to put his coat on, he begins to sway and becomes very pale but starts to sweat; what medical emergency is this?

A Anaphylaxis

B Asthma attack

C Faint

D Myocardial infarction

E Stroke

7 What is the medical condition that causes the muscles of the air passages to go into spasm/narrow, causing wheezing or shortness of breath?

A Asthma

B COPD

C Hyperventilation

D Myocardial infarction

E Stroke

8 You have attended a training day on medical emergencies and first aid, your tutor asks you what ABCDE stands for; which of the following is correct?

A Airway, breathalise, curriculum, disable, expose

B Airway, breathing, circulation, disability, exposure

C Airway, back, circulation, disjointed, exposure

D Airway, breathing, correcting, dysfunction, exploited

E Asthma, breathing, correct, distribution, exhale

9 A parent rushes a child into the surgery from the house across the street; the child has eaten a tube of toothpaste and is not feeling very well. What do you suggest as a first option?

A Give the child copious amounts of milk

B Nothing, the child most likely has a sickness bug

C Send them straight to A&E

D Suggest the mum puts the toothpaste out of reach of the children next time

E Tell the mum to put the child to bed, the child is clearly unwell

10 Which of the following best describes anaphylaxis?

A A medical condition that causes a patient to faint when anxious or nervous.

B A severe allergic reaction that could potentially be life threatening

C A type of stroke

D An allergic reaction to dental materials such as latex or anaesthetic

E An allergic reaction to nuts

Extended Matching Questions

For each of the following questions, select the most appropriate answer from the list below. The answers might be used once, more than once, or not at all.

Topic: Medical Emergencies

a) Anaphylactic shock
b) Angina attack
c) Asthma attack
d) Diabetic hypoglycaemic
e) Hyperventilation
f) Myocardial infarction
g) Tonic–clonic seizure
h) Vasovagal syncope

1   A patient in the dental practice is experiencing a medical emergency. The patient is given chlorphenamine orally. Which of the options listed is the most likely medical condition that this patient is suffering from?

2   A common emergency event in a dental practice is a faint. This can be for many reasons, one of the main reasons is fear or phobia. Which of the options listed is the correct term for a faint?

3   Oxygen cylinders must be kept on the premises at all times, they must be signposted and easily accessible. Which of the conditions listed would you not administer oxygen for?

Answers

1 A patient comes into surgery and says they have a pain in their chest; you check the medical history and it is clear, the patient appears pale but responding well. What do you do?

Correct Answer: b) Make the patient comfortable, ask for help and prepare for Basic Life Support.

If the patient is experiencing chest pain and shows a change in skin colour, you should prepare for Basic Life Support, make the patient comfortable and ask for help.

2 A patient attends the dental practice and hands you an updated medical history; you notice the patient is taking metformin, what condition is this medication used for?

Correct Answer: e) Type 2 diabetes

Metformin is a common drug for patients with type 2 diabetes. This will be prescribed by a doctor or consultant.

3 You are training a member of staff on medical emergencies, when talking about cardiac arrest you explain the CPR ratio. What is the CPR ratio on an adult?

Correct Answer: d) 30:2

The CPR ratio for an adult is 30 compressions to 2 breaths. Pocket masks and BVM can be used if preferred. CPR can now be accompanied by a defibrillator. A defibrillator uses shock patterns when detecting a rhythm on a patient during CPR.

4 A patient who is known for having epilepsy has a seizure while waiting for his exam appointment; before he goes into seizure, which of the following is not a sign for a seizure?

Correct Answer: b) Feeling hungry

The main signs for a seizure are

- loss of consciousness
- rigidity
- convulsive moments
- incontinence
- blank stare
- confusion.

5 During paediatric CPR, how many breaths are given before compressions are started?

Correct Answer: e) 5

Five breaths are given before starting CPR. This is because when a paediatric patient goes into arrest, it can often be respiratory arrest.

6 A patient had a simple extraction of the lower left second molar; it was the last appointment of the day and the patient had come straight from work. As the patient begins to put his coat on, he begins to sway and becomes very pale but starts to sweat. What medical emergency is this?

Correct Answer: c) Faint

If a patient has been at work all day, it could mean they had not eaten before the appointment; therefore, their blood sugars could be low. The signs the patient is showing most likely mean the patient is going to faint. To treat a faint, the best thing to do is to sit or lay them down and elevate the legs; and, if conscious, give oral glucose.

7 What is the medical condition that causes the muscles of the air passages to go into spasm/narrow, causing wheezing or shortness of breath?

Correct Answer: a) Asthma

Asthma is the most common respiratory condition. It is when the muscles of the air passages narrow, which causes symptoms such as: shortness of breath, wheezing, coughing, unconsciousness, and in severe cases even death. This is more commonly known as an asthma attack.

8 You have attended a training day on medical emergencies and first aid; your tutor asks you what ABCDE stands for, which of the following is correct?

Correct Answer: b) Airway, breathing, circulation, disability, exposure

ABCDE (airway, breathing, circulation, disability and exposure) is commonly used to assess a patient that is acutely ill. The patient should be assessed and treated using the principle ABCDE. If there is a deterioration, reassessment should be performed starting at A.

9 A parent rushes a child into the surgery from the house across the street; the child has eaten a tube of toothpaste and is not feeling very well. What do you suggest as a first option?

Correct Answer: a) Give the child copious amounts of milk

In this situation, you can assume the child has overdosed on fluoride. To counteract the fluoride you should give the child large amounts of milk and contact 999.

10 Which of the following best describes anaphylaxis?

Correct Answer: b) A severe allergic reaction that could potentially be life threatening

Anaphylaxis is described as a severe allergic reaction which, if not treated quickly and effectively, could result in death. Anaphylaxis is commonly caused by bee stings, wasp stings, nuts, and latex – although these are not the only causes. During a medical emergency, if a patient is suffering from anaphylactic shock you would treat the patient with adrenaline which may be in the form of an epi pen. It should be administered intramuscularly and 999 should be called.

Extended Matching Questions

For each of the following questions, select the most appropriate answer from the list below. The answers might be used once, more than once, or not at all.

Topic: Medical Emergencies

1   A patient in the dental practice is experiencing a medical emergency. The patient is given chlorphenamine orally. Which of the options listed is the most likely medical condition that this patient is suffering from?

    Correct Answer: a) Anaphylactic shock

    Chlorphenamine is an antihistamine that can be used during an anaphylactic episode. Other drugs commonly used would be adrenaline, hydrocortisone and oxygen. Anaphylactic shock is a serious and potentially life threatening allergic reaction. This type of allergic reaction doesn't always have a sudden onset and, if not treated quickly and accurately, it could become fatal.

2   A common emergency event in a dental practice is a faint. This can be for many reasons, one of the main reasons is fear or phobia. Which of the options listed is the correct term for a faint?

    Correct Answer: h) Vasovagal syncope

    Syncope is the brief loss of consciousness due to a drop in blood pressure. Vasovagal syncope refers to the over activity of the vagus nerve. This results in symptoms such as: pallor, sweating excessively, nausea, and a lowered pulse. It is the reduction of oxygenated blood to the brain that can cause a brief episode of unconsciousness.

3   Oxygen cylinders must be kept on the premises at all times; they must be signposted and easily accessible. Which of the conditions listed would you not administer oxygen for?

    Correct Answer: e) Hyperventilation

    Hyperventilation is rapid breathing that causes a chemical imbalance of carbon dioxide and oxygen in the blood. An episode of hyperventilation is also known as a panic attack. Providing oxygen to a patient suffering with hyperventilation would prolong the emergency.

Further Reading

Levisons textbook for dental nurses by Carole Hollins
GDC standards of the dental team. www.gdc-uk.org/information-standards-guidance
GDC scope of practice. www.gdc-uk.org/scopeofpractice
www.ico.org.uk